Approach to the Patient With a Musculoskeletal Disorder

First Edition

Warren D. Blackburn, Jr, MD

Associate Chief of Staff
for Research and Development
Chief, Rheumatology Section
Birmingham Veteran's Affairs Medical Center
Birmingham, Alabama

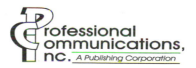

Professional
Communications,
Inc. *A Publishing Corporation*

Published by
Professional Communications, Inc.

For orders, please call
1-800-337-9838

ISBN: 1-884735-38-X

Printed in the United States of America
First Printing, September 1999
Second Printing, March 2000

DISCLAIMER
The opinions expressed in this publication reflect those of the author. However, the author makes no warranty re-garding the contents of the publication. The protocols de-scribed herein are general and may not apply to a specific patient. Any product mentioned in this publication should be taken in accordance with the prescribing information pro-vided by the manufacturer.

This text is printed on recycled paper.

DEDICATION

To Jerry Spenney and YC Parris, whose integrity and
vision exemplify the type of leadership needed to
bring health care into the next millenium. I very
much appreciate their support.

And to my family,
my wife Kathleen,
and my daughters Jennifer, Julia and Laura,
who are the "apples" of their father's eye.

ACKNOWLEDGMENT

I would like to acknowledge the dedication and patience of Malcolm Beasley, Phyllis Freeny and Nikki Weaver.

TABLE OF CONTENTS

TABLES

FIGURES

Introduction

As anyone who has practiced medicine for any time at all knows, medical care is rapidly evolving. On one hand, there have been remarkable, but often expensive, advances in diagnostic techniques (from the clinical laboratory to imaging) and ever improving and targeted therapeutic agents. All too often this has led to overreliance on technology and less attention to a careful history and physical examination.

On the other hand, the emergence of managed care has limited some of the technological reliance and has emphasized cost-effective aspects of care such as the physical examination. Seeing patients with rheumatic diseases remains an area where the history and physical examination are crucial. In fact, this author has seen more referral patients where their primary-care physician was misled by an overreliance on specialized serologies or imaging studies than the other way around. In many of these situations, a simple history and confidence in one's ability to examine the musculoskeletal system would have led to the correct (and it might be added, inexpensively obtained) diagnosis.

This book is intended for the primary-care physician; the emphasis is the diagnosis and treatment of specific rheumatic diseases, but brief sections are included reviewing pathogenesis and occurrence of the specific disorders. The book is not intended to be all inclusive, and many obscure syndromes have been purposely omitted.

Since many patients with musculoskeletal problems present with complaints of "arthritis," as an introduction, it seemed worthwhile to relate an approach which this author has found useful when evaluating such patients.

First, does the patient actually have arthritis? Frequently, soft tissue rheumatism is confused with arthritis. In general, individuals with these disorders have localized pain around the joint and pain is only produced by motions which stress that structure. For example, a patient with olecranon bursitis may only have pain with flexion of the elbow, but pronation and supination may be pain free.

Secondly, is the process inflammatory? Although disorders such as osteoarthritis may have a degree of inflammation, in general these disorders do not manifest the systemic inflammatory signs and symptoms of prototypical inflammatory disorders. Thus fever, weight loss, decreased appetite, fatigue, and prolonged morning stiffness in a patient with a rheumatic disease is more suggestive of rheumatoid arthritis, systemic lupus, infection, or perhaps a vasculitic process than osteoarthritis.

Third, what is the onset and course? Extremely rapid onset of arthritis, within minutes or hours, is indicative of gout. Onset over a day or so may suggest pseudogout, infectious arthritis, or Reiter's syndrome. Rheumatoid arthritis and osteoarthritis usually evolve over longer periods of time.

Fourth, what is the joint distribution? How many joints are involved? Is the distribution symmetrical? Does it involve axial versus peripheral or large versus small joints? A mono- or oligoarthritis may be due to crystal disease, infection, juvenile chronic arthritis, or perhaps a seronegative spondyloarthropathy. Rheumatoid arthritis and lupus are often associated with a symmetrical arthritis. In each chapter, a drawing depicts the more commonly involved joints.

Finally, are there extra-articular features that would be helpful in making the diagnosis? Does the patient have psoriasis, the butterfly rash, or mucosal ulcers seen in lupus? Is the skin thickened, suggestive of scleroderma? Are there tophi or rheumatoid nodules suggestive of gout or rheumatoid arthritis respectively? Answering each of these questions will often limit the differential diagnosis and allow the directed and limited application of imaging studies and laboratory tests.

Ankylosing Spondylitis

The seronegative spondyloarthropathies (SNSAs) represent a group of disorders generally characterized by:

- An asymmetric oligoarthritis
- Spinal involvement
- Somewhat distinctive extra-articular features.

Disorders included under the rubric of SNSA are:

- Ankylosing spondylitis (AS)
- Reiter's syndrome
- Psoriatic arthritis
- Inflammatory-bowel–associated arthritis.

In most of these disorders, there is a remarkable association with the class I histocompatibility human leukocyte antigen (HLA)-B27 and a sharing of certain clinical features. Recognizing this, common criteria have been proposed for the diagnosis of the spondyloarthropathies (Table 1.1). Despite the common features of these disorders, they are distinctive enough to deserve individual consideration.

The first clinical descriptions of AS were from the mid- to late 1800s and variably carried the name of the describing clinicians Marie, Strumpel, and von Bechterew. In the early part of this century, confusion with rheumatoid arthritis led to references as rheumatoid variants or rheumatoid spondylitis. The distinct nature of this disorder was cemented in the 1960s and 1970s by a series of careful epidemiologic studies and the recognition of the association with HLA-B27.

TABLE 1.1 — EUROPEAN SPONDYLARTHROPATHY STUDY GROUP CRITERIA FOR SERONEGATIVE SPONDYLOARTHROPATHIES

Variable	Definition
Inflammatory spinal pain	History or present symptoms of spinal pain in back, dorsal, or cervical region, with at least four of the following: (a) onset before age 45, (b) insidious onset, (c) improved by exercise, (d) associated with morning stiffness, (e) at least 3 months' duration
Synovitis	Past or present asymmetric arthritis, or arthritis predominantly in the lower limbs
Family history	Presence in first-degree or second-degree relatives of any of the following: (a) ankylosing spondylitis, (b) psoriasis, (c) acute uveitis, (d) reactive arthritis, (e) inflammatory bowel disease
Psoriasis	Past or present psoriasis diagnosed by a physician
Inflammatory bowel disease	Past or present Crohn's disease or ulcerative colitis diagnosed by a physician and confirmed by radiographic examination or endoscopy
Alternating buttock pain	Past or present pain alternating between the right and left gluteal regions

Enthesopathy	Past or present spontaneous pain or tenderness at examination of the site of the insertion of the Achilles tendon or plantar fascia
Acute diarrhea	Episode of diarrhea occurring within 1 month before arthritis onset
Urethritis	Nongonococcal urethritis or cervicitis occurring within 1 month before arthritis onset
Sacroiliitis	Bilateral grade 2–4 or unilateral grade 3–4, according to the following radiographic grading system: 0 = normal, 1 = possible, 2 = minimal, 3 = moderate, and 4 = ankylosis

Dougados M, et al. *Arthritis Rheum.* 1991;34:1218-1227.

Pathogenesis

The pathogenesis of the SNSAs is still to be elucidated, but available evidence indicates an association with B27 (in particular subtype 2705) and gastrointestinal (GI) inflammation. In rats that are transgenic for B27, there is inflammation of the GI tract that develops prior to other manifestations of the disease. In humans with AS, colonic inflammation is also frequently found. Of note, certain antibodies to enteric organisms react with B27. However, in rats transgenic for B27 that are raised in germ-free environments, some manifestations of the disease are not apparent. The specific mechanisms that relate gut-associated flora and/or inflammation with B27 are being defined.

Despite the fact that all the risk of developing AS cannot be attributed to B27, recent studies indicate that nearly all of the risk in humans can be associated with genetic susceptibility markers.

Occurrence

The prevalence of the SNSAs varies considerably among various ethnic and racial groups and correlates fairly well with the occurrence of B27 in the population. Of the SNSAs, AS has been best studied. In American whites, it has been estimated that between 0.1% to 0.2% have AS, whereas approximately 8% of normals in this group are B27 positive. In African blacks, where B27 is essentially nonexistent, so is the occurrence of AS. In American blacks, B27 is found in about 2% and the occurrence of AS is much less frequent than in American whites. In northern Norwegians, AS is seen in about 1.4% of the population. The disease is most often recognized in men, who account for approximately 90% of recognized cases of AS.

Clinical features of AS as shown in Table 1.2 include:

- Back pain as the presenting symptom
- Symptoms initially occurring during adolescence or early adulthood (later onset is distinctively unusual)
- Pain, ranging from mild to severe and is:
  - Persistent
  - Generally deep and aching
  - Poorly localized to the buttocks or low lumbar area.

TABLE 1.2 — CLINICAL FEATURES OF ANKYLOSING SPONDYLITIS

- Back pain, particularly in a young male
- Prolonged morning stiffness
- Improvement with exercise
- Enthesopathy
- Extra-articular involvement, especially iritis

Back discomfort and stiffness usually worsens after periods of inactivity and is particularly worse on arising in the morning. Pain usually abates somewhat with motion or exercise.

The extent of axial involvement is variable and many patients will have evidence of sacroiliitis without further involvement or limitation. An occasional patient will have progressive disease with involvement of the entire axial skeleton, ultimately leading to spinal fusion and its attendant disability (Figure 1.1). In these cases, thoracic and cervical pain will usually be noted. Although pain can continue for many years, some patients note pain remission with fusion of the axial skeleton.

FIGURE 1.1 — PATIENT WITH SPINAL FUSION OF ANKYLOSING SPONDYLITIS

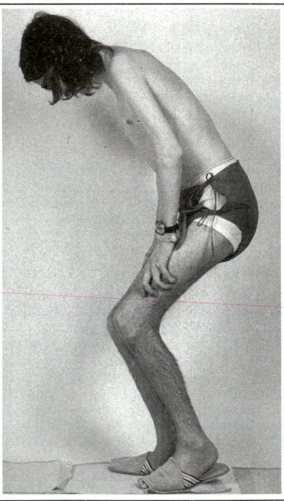

A young man with advanced ankylosing spondylitis with essentially complete fusion of the axial skeleton.

Courtesy of Syntex Laboratories, Inc.

In most cases of AS, axial symptoms predominate; however, some patients will note extra-axial joint involvement that can be associated with significant disability (Figure 1.2). Adolescents, in particular, may have involvement of the hips or, less frequently, the shoulders. Often this involvement is symmetrical. Other patients with AS may have an asymmetric oligoarthritis involving the knee or other lower extremity joint.

Enthesopathy, or inflammation at ligament or tendon insertion sites, is frequently observed in patients with AS. Typical locations include:
- Achilles' tendon (Figure 1.3)
- Ischial and tibial tuberosities
- Plantar fascial attachment sites.

Extra-articular features occur in the minority of patients with AS, but can be devastating. About 25% of patients with AS will have anterior uveitis, which is the most common extra-articular feature of the disease. In most, this is unilateral and is characterized by remissions and often widely spaced exacerbations. Patients notice blurred vision, increased lacrimation, eye pain and photophobia. On slit lamp examination, cells usually are seen in the anterior chamber.

Even in those patients who have ankylosis of the thoracic spine, pulmonary involvement is rare. Some do develop apical fibrosis. Generally, this is an asymptomatic finding noted on a chest radiograph. The lesion can become cavitary and secondarily colonized with fungi (such as *Aspergillus*) or with bacteria. In those situations, cough and hemoptysis may develop.

A few patients with AS will develop inflammation of the ascending aorta resulting in dilatation of the root and aortic insufficiency. Similar changes may be seen in the conducting system, interfering with cardiac rhythm. Interestingly, B27 has been linked to

FIGURE 1.2 — DIAGRAM DEPICTING JOINT INVOLVEMENT IN ANKYLOSING SPONDYLITIS

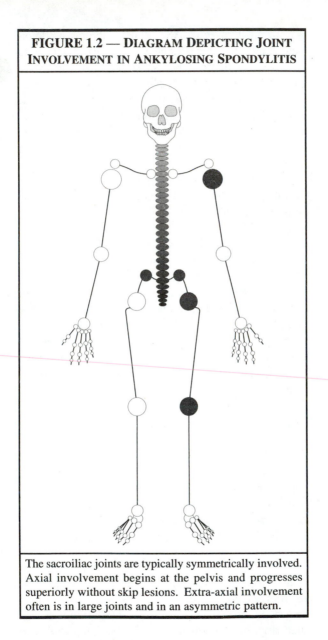

The sacroiliac joints are typically symmetrically involved. Axial involvement begins at the pelvis and progresses superiorly without skip lesions. Extra-axial involvement often is in large joints and in an asymmetric pattern.

FIGURE 1.3 — SWOLLEN ACHILLES TENDON

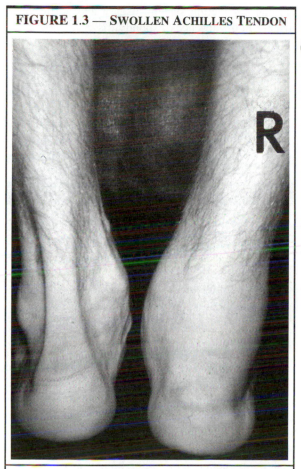

Marked swelling of the right Achilles tendon, typically seen in one of the seronegative spondyloarthropathies.

cardiac conduction system disease and aortic valve disease in the absence of spondylitis.

Patients who have extensive syndesmophytes can develop cord compression and symptoms of spinal stenosis. In those who have back and hip involvement, it can be difficult to sort out the source of the symptoms until neurological deficits occur.

Finally, amyloidosis has been reported in the rare case of AS, but should be considered in a patient who develops proteinuria.

Laboratory Tests and Radiographs

Ankylosing spondylitis is an inflammatory disorder and laboratory tests reflect this fact:

- Acute phase reactants are elevated, as may be white blood cell and platelet counts.
- Serum immunoglobulin A (IgA) levels may be elevated in some patients.
- B27 is present in about 90% of patients.

Radiographs are most useful in defining the disease. Sacroiliitis is bilateral in patients with AS and is recognized initially as haziness of the margins of the sacroiliac joints (Figure 1.4). Over time, erosions become apparent, which may give the impression that the joint space is actually widened. Sclerosis and ultimately fusion of the joint follow this finding. Other imaging procedures, including bone scans, computed tomography and magnetic resonance imaging may increase sensitivity, but this comes with some loss of specificity. Few clinical situations require these tests to aid in the diagnosis.

Squaring of the vertebral bodies occurs due to inflammation at attachment sites of the annulus fibrosis to the body (Figure 1.5). Later, ossification occurs with the formation of syndesmophytes, or vertical bony bridges that can be differentiated from the hori-

FIGURE 1.4 — RADIOGRAPHS OF THE SACROILIAC JOINT

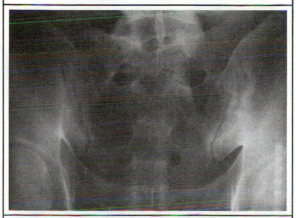

An anteroposterior radiograph of the pelvis demonstrating sclerosis and erosions with pseudo-widening of the sacroiliac joints.

Courtesy of Arthritis Foundation.

zontal osteophyte. Chronic enthesopathic changes can be seen as bony whiskering and are likely to be seen at attachment sites around the pelvis and knee (Figure 1.6). Radiographs of involved hips may demonstrate concentric cartilage loss and the exuberant bone formation may lead to fusion.

Diagnosis

The diagnosis of AS is most readily made by eliciting symptoms of back pain which have characteristics of an inflammatory disorder in a young man and demonstrate characteristic radiographic features. Criteria have been developed and are listed in Table 1.1. Once sacroiliitis has been demonstrated radiographically, the differential diagnosis is limited (apart from the SNSAs), but should include infection and other

FIGURE 1.5 — AXIAL SKELETON SHOWING SQUARING

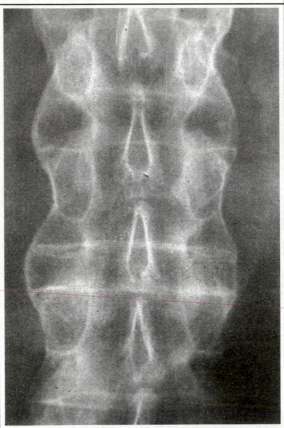

Radiographs of the axial skeleton demonstrating the flowing syndesmophytes typical of ankylosing spondylitis. Note that disc height is preserved.

Courtesy of Arthritis Foundation.

FIGURE 1.6 — WHISKERING X-RAY

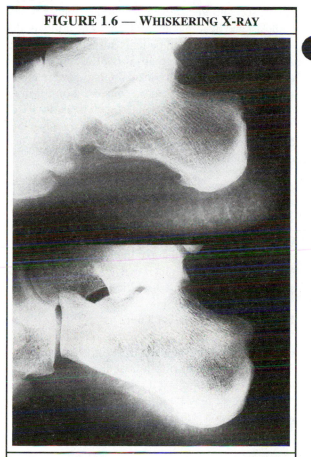

Radiograph of the calcaneus from a patient with a serone-gative spondyloarthropathy demonstrating whiskering at the insertion of the longitudinal ligament and erosive changes at the Achilles tendon insertion site.

Courtesy of Arthritis Foundation.

readily recognized disorders, including paraplegia, sarcoidosis, and hyperparathyroidism. The utility of determining B27 status in patients suspected of having AS is controversial. Perhaps it is of use in high-risk patients or patients with back pain who have relatives with AS. Regardless of these considerations, it must be remembered that despite the fact that about 8% of American whites have B27, but only 0.1% have AS, demonstrates the lack of specificity of this test when used in isolation.

Management

Ankylosing spondylitis has no known cure and there is no evidence that medical intervention decreases the extent of the axial skeleton involvement. Nonetheless, there is much that can be done to preserve function and limit disability.

■ Nonpharmacological Therapy

A stretching and exercise program is useful in maintaining muscle strength and limiting deformity. Simple modifications of activities may also be important in limiting deformity. For example, use of a small pillow at night may limit the degree of cervical flexion and, if fusion is to occur, to have it occur in a functional position.

■ Pharmacological Therapy

Pharmacological therapy usually involves nonsteroidal anti-inflammatory drugs (NSAIDs). Used at full anti-inflammatory doses, they are quite useful in limiting pain during periods of disease activity. Symptoms due to an enthesopathy may be well treated with NSAIDs or with local instillation of corticosteroids. Systemic steroids are usually of no use in treating the axial or articular features of this disease. Sulfasalazine, particularly in doses of at least 2000 mg/d, may

26

be useful in selected patients with axial disease. Both sulfasalazine and methotrexate have been used successfully to treat the extra-axial arthritis. Eye involvement is usually treated with mydriatics and/or topical steroids.

SUGGESTED READING

Arnett F. Ankylosing spondylitis. In: Koopman WJ, ed. *Arthritis and Allied Conditions*: *A Textbook of Rheumatology*. 13th ed. Baltimore, Md; Williams and Wilkins; 1996:1197-1208.

Clegg DO, Reda DJ, Weisman MH, et al. Comparison of sulfasalazine and placebo in the treatment of ankylosing spondylitis. A Department of Veterans Affairs Cooperative Study. *Arthritis Rheum*. 1996;39:2004-2012.

Dougados M, van der Linden S, Juhlin R, et al. The European Spondylarthropathy Study Group preliminary criteria for the classification of spondyloarthropathy. *Arthritis Rheum*. 1991;34:1218-1227.

Gran JT. An epidemiologic survey of the signs and symptoms of ankylosing spondylitis. *Clin Rheumatol*. 1985;4:161-169.

Arthritis Associated With Inflammatory Bowel Disease

The arthritis associated with Crohn's disease and ulcerative colitis:

- Is associated with the expression of human leukocyte antigen (HLA)-B27
- Has a prominent axial component
- Has a distinctive peripheral arthritis
- Occurs in the absence of rheumatoid factor.

As such, the arthritis associated with these inflammatory bowel diseases (IBDs) is considered as a disorder under the rubric of the seronegative spondyloarthropathies (SNSAs).

Pathogenesis

Despite the clinical association between gut inflammation and arthritis, the mechanisms that result in the development of arthritis are still not understood. However, postulated mechanisms consider that the increased mucosal permeability leads to less filtered release of gut luminal antigens. Further, the expression of DR on epithelial cells and accumulation of $CD4^+$ T cells have led to speculation that luminal antigens may generate an amplified response rather than inducing tolerance. Potentially, a number of antigens apart from an undefined initiating one could account for disease exacerbations.

Occurrence

The prevalence of IBD varies depending upon ethnic and racial distributions. It appears to occur more often in whites than in individuals of color. Those with Jewish ancestry have a higher prevalence. In the general population, the prevalence of IBD is about 150 per 100,000. Of course, most will not have arthritis but, of these 10% to 20% will develop the disease.

Clinical Features

The arthritis associated with IBD may be peripheral and/or axial. The peripheral involvement is typically an oligoarticular asymmetric arthritis (Figure 2.1). Clinical features include:
- Joints most often involved are in the lower extremity, but may be either small or large joints
- Periods of exacerbations and remissions
- Usually, no erosive changes seen
- Occurrence after or coincidental with the gut disease in ulcerative colitis.

There is an association between the extent of colonic disease in either ulcerative colitis or Crohn's disease and peripheral arthritis, but small bowel involvement and Crohn's disease are not associated.

In contrast to ankylosing spondylitis (AS), axial involvement associated with IBD is seen as often in women as in men. Women may have an earlier onset and more severe disease. The clinical presentation may be identical to that seen in patients with AS and includes:
- Low back pain
- Stiffness
- Limitations of motion
- Axial involvement preceding the bowel disease (symptoms are unrelated to the degree of bowel disease)
- Finding of B27 in about one third of individuals with IBD and axial involvement.

FIGURE 2.1 — DIAGRAM DEPICTING JOINT INVOLVEMENT IN INFLAMMATORY BOWEL DISEASE

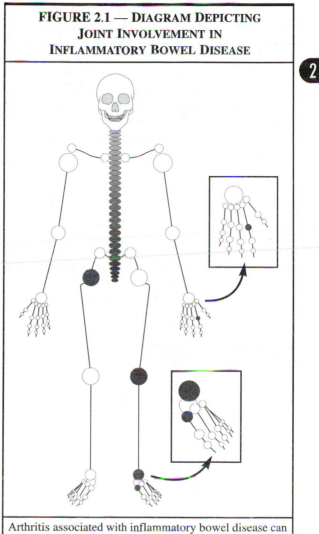

Arthritis associated with inflammatory bowel disease can be either axial or, when there is extra-axial involvement, it tends to be oligoarticular, particularly involving the noted joints.

Interestingly, in a prospective evaluation of patients with AS, those who were B27–negative were more likely to develop IBD than those who carried this marker.

Enthesopathy, similar to other SNSAs, is a part of the illness associated with IBD. Clubbing of the digits is also occasionally seen as another skeletal manifestation of these disorders.

The predominant extra-articular features of IBD are those related to the gut. Classic symptoms include:

- Abdominal pain
- Weight loss
- Diarrhea.

Skin findings may be as common as articular changes. Erythema nodosum may occur and parallel the course of the bowel disease, whereas the less common pyoderma gangrenosum does not. Anterior uveitis is seen particularly in those who have axial involvement and are B27–positive.

Laboratory Tests and Radiographs

The laboratory features of arthritis associated with inflammatory bowel disease are mostly those related to the acute phase response. Erythrocyte sedimentation rate and C-reactive protein are elevated. There may be anemia of chronic disease, which may be exacerbated by gastrointestinal (GI) blood loss.

Radiographs of peripheral joints may reveal soft tissue swelling but, as noted above, erosions are unusual. When the axial skeleton is involved, findings on radiographs may be indistinguishable from those seen in AS.

Diagnosis

In patients with known IBD, the diagnosis of the associated arthritis is not difficult (Table 2.1). On a rare occasion, arthritis may be a direct complication of IBD or its treatment. Patients with intestinal perforation may seed a nearby hip. Similarly, patients treated with corticosteroids for their bowel disease may develop aseptic necrosis of the hip, which may be confused with an inflammatory arthritis. Patients with diarrhea or other GI symptoms and arthritis, but who have not been evaluated and found to have IBD, may actually suffer from a number of other, different disorders.

TABLE 2.1 — OTHER DIAGNOSES TO ACCOUNT FOR ARTHRITIS IN PATIENTS WITH INFLAMMATORY BOWEL DISEASE

- Septic arthritis
- Avascular necrosis
- Crystal-induced arthritis

Ankylosing spondylitis or reactive arthritis related to dysentery are part of the differential diagnosis. Whipple's disease may present with arthritis that is usually transient, but may become chronic and precede symptoms suggestive of bowel disease by several years. In those symptoms, the characteristic histology and evidence of infection with *Tropheryma whippelii* are helpful in delineating the disorders. Patients with jejunal-ileal bypass often have a baseline diarrhea. They may develop an episodic illness characterized by fever and migratory arthritis. Often this disorder is responsive to antibiotics; however, it is sometimes persistent enough that reversal of the bypass becomes necessary.

Management

The peripheral arthritis may respond to whatever therapy is needed to treat the underlying bowel disease. If additional therapy is needed, frequently nonsteroidal anti-inflammatory drugs (NSAIDs) are sufficient, but many patients with IBD cannot tolerate NSAIDs. Sulfasalazine is useful in treating the peripheral arthritis and the underlying bowel disease. Intra-articular injections with corticosteroids are often useful in patients with mono- or oligoarticular disease, but systemic corticosteroids are rarely needed to treat the arthritis. Colonic resection, particularly in ulcerative colitis, often improves the peripheral articular disease.

The course of the axial disease generally does not parallel the bowel disease. Therapy is the same as for a patient with isolated AS. Here as well, NSAIDs are often used successfully, but many patients are intolerant of full anti-inflammatory doses.

SUGGESTED READING

Gravallese E, Kantrowitz FG. Arthritic manifestations of inflammatory bowel disease. *Am J Gastroenterol.* 1988;83:703-709.

Greenstein A, Janowitz HD, Sachar DB. The extraintestinal complications of Crohn's disease and ulcerative colitis: a study of 700 patients. *Medicine.* 1976;55:401-412.

Scarpa R, del Puente A, D'Arienzo A, et al. The arthritis of ulcerative colitis: clinical and genetic aspects. *J Rheumatol.* 1992;19: 373-377.

Stein HB, Schlappner OL, Boyko W, Gourlay RH, Reeve CE. The intestinal bypass: arthritis-dermatitis syndrome. *Arthritis Rheum.* 1981;24:684-690.

3

Calcium Crystal Disorders

Soon after the observation was made that mono-sodium urate crystals were responsible for gout, it became apparent that some patients had a disorder that was similar in its clinical presentation to acute gout, but urate crystals could not be found in the synovial fluid. Further examination of the fluids from these patients led to the discovery of crystals that were found to be composed of calcium pyrophosphate dihydrate (CPPD). Based on the similarities of the clinical presentation of these patients and those with gout, the term pseudogout was established. Subsequently, a number of clinical presentations have been ascribed to these crystals. Additionally, a number of other calcium crystals have been found and linked to human disease.

Pathogenesis

The mechanisms responsible for formation of CPPD crystals in the joint are not fully elucidated and may be multifactorial. The crystals interact with cartilage matrix, and it has been suggested that alterations in the matrix promote crystal formation. Alternatively, changes in the concentration of calcium or pyrophosphate may also promote crystal formation. Several metabolic alterations have been invoked to account for this finding. It seems likely that, as with many things in medicine, each of these may play a role; the most important one in any given individual may be different.

Regardless of the mechanism that results in crystal formation, CPPD crystals:

- Induce an inflammatory response
- Activate, complement and trigger neutrophil production of leukotrienes and other inflammatory molecules
- Stimulate proliferation of synovial cells and induce release of cytokines from mononuclear phagocytes, although they are much less potent than urate crystals.

Occurrence

To a large extent, the prevalence of disease associated with crystals of CPPD is not known. Even in centers attuned to the diagnosis of crystal-induced disease, patients admitted with acute arthritis due to CPPD are about 50% as common as those admitted with gout. On the other hand, evidence of cartilage calcification which often is presumed to be due to CPPD is common. In a series of octogenarians and their elders, nearly half had radiographic evidence of cartilage calcification. Of course, not all had disease which could be attributed to this accumulation of crystals.

Overall, patients with arthritis associated with CPPD tend to be older. In one study, the mean age of patients with CPPD was 72 years. There may be a modestly larger incidence of CPPD-related disorders in men than in women, but the results are not consistent.

Most studies have evaluated these sporadic cases of CPPD deposition disease, but important associations have also been noted with certain metabolic diseases (see *Diagnosis*, this chapter). Further, a definite familial association of unusually early onset CPPD deposition disease has been noted. In these families, the severity of the disease has been variable, but most are thought to have autosomal dominant inheritance patterns. Specific genetic characteristics related to the development of familial disease have not been determined.

Clinical Presentation

It has been long recognized that CPPD crystals are responsible for a number of clinical presentations in addition to the best recognized one, pseudogout.

Pseudogout is generally an acute illness. It represents about 25% of symptomatic patients with CPPD deposition disease, but this may be an overrepresentation as it is the most readily diagnosed form of the disorder. Like its namesake, patients with pseudogout will often report, prior to the diagnostic attack, "petite" episodes or short-duration, low-severity episodes. Often, no clear precipitating event can be determined, but major surgery, trauma or medical illnesses have been linked to acute attacks. Changes in fluid and electrolyte balance are common, which may alter crystal solubility in the joint. Development of pseudogout after a functioning parathyroid adenoma is removed is a well described event.

The attack of pseudogout will occur abruptly and reach its peak intensity in hours to days, at times raising the question of septic arthritis. The knee joint is most often involved, but the shoulders, elbows, ankles, wrists and first metatarsophalangeal may also be affected (Figure 3.1). At times, patients will present with a cluster of joints that are simultaneously or sequentially involved. The joints are often warm, swollen and mildly erythematous. Typically, the signs and symptoms will resolve in days to weeks.

Perhaps the most common presentation related to crystals of CPPD is that of a degenerative arthritis or pseudo-osteoarthritis. It involves the knees, wrists, elbows, ankles, and metacarpophalangeals (MCPs). Some patients will report occasional episodes of acute arthritis, but others may simply have pain and mild

37

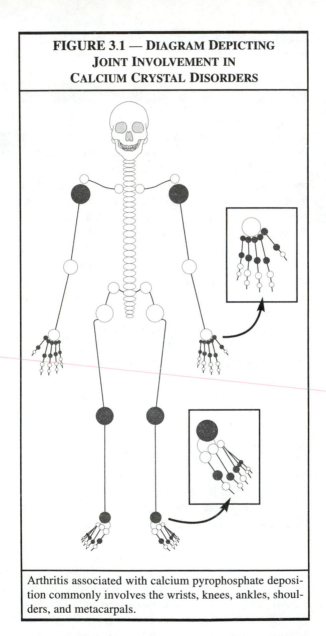

FIGURE 3.1 — DIAGRAM DEPICTING JOINT INVOLVEMENT IN CALCIUM CRYSTAL DISORDERS

Arthritis associated with calcium pyrophosphate deposition commonly involves the wrists, knees, ankles, shoulders, and metacarpals.

effusions. When there is involvement of joints typical for osteoarthritis, the diagnosis of CPPD deposition disease may be overlooked. Involvement of joints atypical for osteoarthritis, a history of intermittent acute attacks, and demonstration of chondrocalcinosis on plain radiographs should suggest the diagnosis.

A third presentation which may cause some diagnostic and therapeutic confusion is pseudorheumatoid arthritis. These patients may have a symmetrical small joint polyarthritis and some will have rheumatoid factor in their serum, usually of low titer. The prognosis is generally good and patients tend not to have erosive changes on radiographs of the hands.

Some patients also have accumulation of CPPD crystal in the axial skeleton and the disorder is occasionally confused with ankylosing spondylitis. True bony ankylosis is not part of this syndrome.

Laboratory Findings and Radiographs

The most characteristic laboratory feature in CPPD deposition disease is the demonstration of crystals in synovial fluid. The crystals are positively birefringent (Figure 3.2). They are shorter and less bright under polarized light than monosodium urate crystals, but may also be found intra-cellularly. Synovial fluid from patients with CPPD deposition disease is characteristically inflammatory. White blood cell counts are elevated and most are neutrophils.

Other laboratory tests are nonspecific. Acute phase proteins may be elevated during an acute attack. Laboratory tests may reflect an associated medical condition such as hyperparathyroidism or hemochromatosis.

Radiographs may reveal calcifications in cartilage and ligaments that frequently are stippled or linear (Figure 3.3). Calcification is often observed in:

- The triangular cartilage of the wrist

FIGURE 3.2 — POLARIZED LIGHT SHOWING CALCIUM PYROPHOSPHATE DIHYDRATE CRYSTAL NEXT TO URIC ACID CRYSTAL

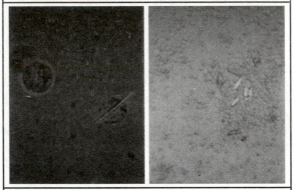

Left: The negatively birefringent crystal of monosodium urate. Right: In contrast, the smaller, less bright, positively birefringent calcium pyrophosphate dihydrate (CPPD) crystals.

Courtesy of Arthritis Foundation.

- The symphysis pubis
- The shoulder
- Meniscus of the knee.

Additionally, changes consistent with osteoarthritis, although in atypical joints, may be seen in association with CPPD.

Diagnosis

The diagnosis of CPPD deposition disease (Table 3.1) is most often considered in a patient with acute mono- or oligoarthritis. Differential diagnosis should include:
- Gout
- Occasionally, septic arthritis
- Perhaps the seronegative spondyloarthropathies (especially Reiter's syndrome).

FIGURE 3.3 — RADIOGRAPH OF THE KNEE DEMONSTRATING CHONDROCALCINOSIS

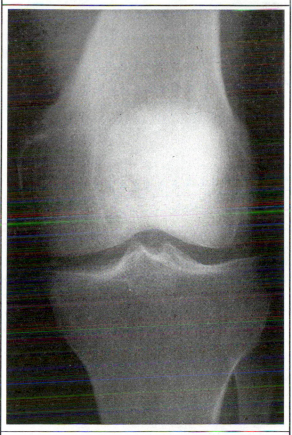

Courtesy of Syntex Laboratories, Inc.

TABLE 3.1 — DIFFERENTIAL DIAGNOSIS OF CALCIUM PYROPHOSPHATE DIHYDRATE

- Benign course
- General lack of extra-articular features
- Joints involved
- Synovial fluid findings

Demonstration of weakly positively birefringent crystals in the synovial fluid serves to confirm the diagnosis.

Symptoms consistent with osteoarthritis (with or without acute episodes) where the involvement is in an atypical joint, such as the shoulder or wrist, should raise suspicions that CPPD may be involved. Confirmation of the diagnosis can again be made by:

- Examining synovial fluid
- Characteristic radiographic findings.

Once the diagnosis of CPPD deposition disease is made, it is generally recommended that disorders which have been associated with these crystals be considered. Both hyperparathyroidism and hemochromatosis have been linked to CPPD disease. Although no formal and controlled epidemiological associations have been made, about 10% of case series of patients with CPPD disease have hyperparathyroidism. Certainly, prolonged hypercalcemia based on the present understanding of crystal formation would be considered a risk factor for the development of CPPD crystals. Based on these observations, it would seem prudent to obtain a serum calcium level and pursue a diagnostic evaluation if elevated.

Similarly, about 50% of the patients with hemochromatosis have arthritis, and a similar fraction have chondrocalcinosis. Findings of arthritis involving the second and third MCPs are also suggestive of the arthritis associated with hemochromatosis.

A number of other disorders, including metabolic disorders resulting in hypomagnesemia, hypophosphatasia, hypothyroidism, Wilson's disease, and ochronosis, have been the subject of case reports linking them to CPPD disease. Although an association has not been proven with epidemiologic study, some of these may be considered from a teleologic perspective. Thus, it would seem reasonable to obtain serum chemistries, iron studies, and thyroid function tests on patients who are found to have CPPD deposition disease, given the relatively low cost of the tests.

Management

Therapy of CPPD deposition disease is divided into prophylactic and acute phases. Unlike gout, there are no medications that have been shown to prevent the disease. Attacks of pseudogout can be controlled with:

- Nonsteroidal anti-inflammatory drugs (NSAIDs)
- Intra-articular corticosteroids
- Intravenous or oral colchicine.

Both NSAIDs and oral colchicine can be used as prophylactic agents.

When CPPD deposition disease presents with an osteoarthritis-like picture, therapy is essentially the same as with osteoarthritis. Pharmacological therapy with acetaminophen is used initially and NSAIDs may be useful for acute attacks or for recalcitrant disease.

In those patients who present with arthritis who are then found to have hemochromatosis, chelating therapy may inhibit the development of complications in other organ systems, but established CPPD deposition disease may proceed.

Other Crystals

It has been long recognized that a number of other calcium crystals are deposited in various locations. Many of these crystals, including hydroxyapatite crystals, are basic calcium phosphate crystals. As a group, they are too small to be seen using routine or polarized optical microscopy, although with certain stains (such as alizarin red S), they can be seen with plain microscopy.

These crystals can be seen radiographically amassed in certain tendons, such as the supraspinatus tendon. They have been associated with an acute or calcific tendinitis. These occur more often in women and may be associated with warmth and erythema.

More recently, several syndromes characterized by arthritis, usually of one or two joints and named after the location where they were described, have been associated with basic calcium phosphate crystals. Milwaukee shoulder is an example. It is seen more often in women and is characterized by:

- Disruption of the rotator cuff
- Resorption of the articular cartilage
- A relatively acellular synovial fluid.

Characterization of the fluid demonstrated large amounts of proteolytic enzymes, including collagenase.

A similar syndrome involving the thumb has been termed the Missouri thumb. In both, basic calcium phosphate salts have been demonstrated. Therapy is generally ineffective and centers around symptomatic interventions.

SUGGESTED READING

Kohn NN, Hughes RE, McCarty DJ, Faires JS. The significance of calcium phosphate crystals in the synovial fluid of arthritis patients: the pseudogout syndrome. II. Identification of crystals. *Ann Intern Med*. 1962;56:738-745.

McCarty DJ. Diagnostic mimicry in arthritis: patterns of joint involvement associated with calcium pyrophosphate dihydrate crystal disease. *Bull Rheum Dis*. 1975;25:804-809.

McCarty DJ, Kohn NN, Faires JS. The significance of calcium phosphate crystals in the synovial fluid of arthritis patients: the psuedogout syndrome. I. Clinical aspects. *Ann Intern Med*. 1962;56:711-737.

Resnick D, Niwayama G, Goergen TG, et al. Clinical, radiographic and pathologic abnormalities in calcium pyrophosphate dihydrate deposition disease (CPPD): pseudogout. *Radiology*. 1977;122:1-15.

3

4 Fibromyalgia

Fibromyalgia is not an inflammatory disorder. Based upon numerous studies evaluating present or previous histories of anxiety and depression, many authors have categorized it as an affective system disorder. Nonetheless, because of the frequency and, at times, severity of the musculoskeletal complaints, patients are frequently seen by physicians with an interest in arthritis and related diseases. It is important to recognize this syndrome, not only to direct appropriate therapy, but also to interdict unnecessary testing.

Pathogenesis

An impressive array of studies have been performed in an attempt to delineate a peripheral mechanism to account for the symptoms of fibromyalgia. Apart from findings from nuclear magnetic resonance spectroscopy indicating a decreased capacity for muscle work and consistent studies demonstrating decreased level of physical fitness, these studies have been negative.

In contrast, a number of studies have demonstrated that many patients with fibromyalgia have a history of:

- Anxiety
- Depressive disorders
- Disordered sleep.

Although not uniformly reproduced, a disruption of nonrapid eye movement sleep with intrusion of alpha waves has been demonstrated.

It has also been shown that plasma cortisol levels are elevated in patients with fibromyalgia, an observation also noted in patients with depression. Further, the peptide substance P levels are increased in the spinal fluid of patients with fibromyalgia. Recent work with single photon emission computed tomographic imaging of the brain has discovered that regional blood flow to the caudate and thalamic nuclei is decreased in patients with fibromyalgia when compared with healthy controls. Interestingly, blood flow to these areas is also decreased in patients with other disorders associated with chronic pain.

Numerous studies have placed a stressful life event prior to the onset of fibromyalgia. These have included:

- Major medical illnesses
- Trauma
- Divorce
- Menopause.

How each of these play a role in the development of the syndrome known as fibromyalgia has not been delineated.

Occurrence

Fibromyalgia is not an unusual condition, although the incidence and prevalence have not been fully ascertained. Estimates of its prevalence in women have ranged up to 13%. Recently, in a study from Kansas, 2% of all women and 5% of women over 65 were thought to have fibromyalgia (Wolfe et al, 1995). The diagnosis is made less often in men. In some studies, over 90% of patients with fibromyalgia are women. The Kansas study found the prevalence in women to be about seven times that in men.

Onset of fibromyalgia is typically in middle age, but it has been reported in children and in elderly adults.

Clinical Presentation

The history given by a patient with fibromyalgia is often distinctive:

- Widespread pain that is localized to specific areas at times
- Extreme fatigue that interferes with many or all activities
- Perceived limited ability to exercise
- Do not feel rested upon waking in the morning
- Diffuse stiffness that may not resolve throughout the day
- Diffuse joint or hand swelling is often described (which cannot be confirmed on physical examination)
- Exacerbation of symptoms upon weather changes and psychological stress.

Although musculoskeletal symptoms are most prominent, patients with fibromyalgia may report a myriad of complaints, reflected in multiple positive responses to a review of systems. Commonly reported symptoms by patients with fibromyalgia are shown in Table 4.1.

Despite the myriad and severity of the complaints, findings on physical examination are usually limited. Specific areas of trigger point tenderness are noted (see *Diagnosis,* this chapter). Joints are not swollen. Despite complaints of weakness, muscle strength testing is normal or will demonstrate give-way weakness. Oral mucosa may be dry due to mouth breathing or anxiety. Rashes usually are not present or simply show evidence of excoriation.

TABLE 4.1 — SYMPTOMS OF FIBROMYALGIA

- Tension or migraine headaches
- Various (often evanescent) rashes
- Photosensitivity
- Dry eyes or mouth
- Hair loss
- Urinary frequency and urgency
- Irritable bowel syndrome
- Extremity paresthesias
- Temporal mandibular joint syndrome
- Weakness
- Dysphagia
- Mucosal ulcers

Laboratory Tests and Radiographs

There are no routine laboratory or radiographic tests whose abnormal findings would indicate fibromyalgia. In fact, abnormal findings reflect either the normal variation in the population or another condition.

Diagnosis

The diagnosis of fibromyalgia is readily made based on the history and physical examination. Indeed, the description is often distinctive enough that, within a few moments of taking a history, the diagnosis is evident. Nonetheless, the American College of Rheumatology has developed diagnostic criteria (Table 4.2). These include a history of widespread pain lasting for at least 3 months with pain on the left and right side of the body and above and below the waist. Additionally, eleven of the eighteen trigger points will be tender with palpation (Figure 4.1).

Apart from a complete history and examination, little or nothing additional is needed to make the di-

TABLE 4.2 — CLASSIFICATION CRITERIA FOR FIBROMYALGIA

- Widespread pain, lasting at least 3 months over all of the following:
  - Left and right side of body
  - Above and below waist
  - Axially, such as C spine, anterior chest, low back or thoracic spine
- Pain over at least 11 of 18 tender points on palpation performed with about 4 kg of force (enough to blanche a fingernail)

Wolfe F, et al. *Arthritis Rheum.* 1990;33:160-172.

agnosis. Thyroid disease and other causes of sleep disorders (sleep apnea or disruptive sleep schedules) may be uncovered in the history and occasionally can be confused or associated with fibromyalgia. Severe depression or other stressful events may provide clues to events that may exacerbate the symptoms.

The finding of normal serum chemistries, blood counts, and perhaps thyroid function tests is reassuring. Certainly, findings of joint swelling or other objective findings may lead to other tests and diagnoses. Lacking objective findings, blood tests to evaluate the presence of autoantibodies are not only unhelpful, but are frequently confusing to the patient and physician. Such confusion has led to inappropriate labeling with terms such as undifferentiated or atypical connective tissue disease.

Perhaps because of the diffuse nature of the complaints, many other tests, including expensive scans, endoscopic procedures, and catheterizations, are at times performed on patients with fibromyalgia. Not only are they usually not warranted, but are expensive and potentially harmful.

FIGURE 4.1 — TRIGGER POINTS OF FIBROMYALGIA

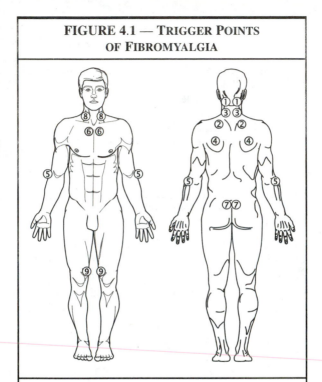

Specific tender points seen in patients with fibromyalgia are: 1) Suboccipital muscle insertion into the occiput; 2) Midpoint of the trapezial ridge; 3) Anterior aspect of the neck between C5 and C7; 4) Medial and superior to the scapula; 5) Distal to the lateral epicondyle; 6) The costochondral junction of the second rib; 7) Lumbar spine at the upper border of the buttock; 8) Posterior to the trochanteric bursa; 9) Medial fat pad of the knee, proximal to the joint space.

Management

Treatment of patients with fibromyalgia is often time consuming. Distraught after being subjected to numerous tests, most patients find that conviction alone on the part of the physician that the diagnosis is correct is often consoling. Many patients will indicate their relief that they are not believed to be manufacturing their symptoms. Being informed that fibromyalgia does not result in muscle or joint damage or deformity is also reassuring.

■ Nonpharmacological Therapy

Perhaps the most successful therapy for fibromyalgia is an aerobic conditioning program. As noted above, most patients with fibromyalgia are deconditioned. Prescriptions for exercise, however, are often met with resistance and complaints that it exacerbates symptoms. Nonetheless, aerobic exercise:

- Does produce improvement in rating of physical function
- Improves sleep
- Has the benefits of cardiovascular conditioning.

Pool exercises seem to be well accepted and tolerated by most fibromyalgia patients and have the advantage of upper- and lower-extremity exercise. Choice of the aerobic exercise is left to the patient to encourage compliance. Those who choose walking or bicycling may want to add an upper-extremity weight program.

■ Pharmacological Therapy

Pharmacological therapy is helpful to reestablish a more normal sleep pattern. Perhaps best studied is the tricyclic antidepressant amitriptyline. Its soporific effects are useful when administered nocturnally and it has been shown to decrease reports of pain and improve sleep. Moreover, this medication is helpful in the patient who has underlying depression. In some, the response to amitriptyline wanes with time, and this may be reversed with dosage adjustments.

Cyclobenzaprine also has been shown to be effective in treatment of fibromyalgia. Interestingly, serotonin reuptake inhibitors have not been shown to be more effective than placebo; perhaps this is related to the fact that they often are less soporific.

Many patients are treated with nonsteroidal anti-inflammatory drugs, presumably because of their musculoskeletal complaints. However, they have not been shown to be more effective than placebo in treatment of fibromyalgia. Nonetheless, patients frequently will continue to request and use analgesic medication. In those circumstances, recommendations for acetaminophen may be useful and will alleviate concerns regarding gastrointestinal irritation or risk of habituation with narcotics.

SUGGESTED READING

Carette S, Bell MJ, Reynolds WJ, et al. Comparison of amitriptyline, cyclobenzaprine, and placebo in the treatment of fibromyalgia. A randomized double-blind clinical trial. *Arthritis Rheum*. 1994;37:32-40.

Moldofsky H. Sleep and fibrositis syndrome. *Rheum Dis Clin North Am*. 1989;15:91-103.

Moldofsky H, Scarisbrick P, England R, Smythe H. Musculoskeletal symptoms and non-REM sleep disturbance in patients with "fibrositis" syndrome and healthy subjects. *Psychosom Med*. 1975; 37:341-351.

Wolfe F, Ross K, Anderson J, Russell IJ, Hebert L. The prevalence and characteristics of fibromyalgia in the general population. *Arthritis Rheum*. 1995;38:19-28.

Wolfe F, Smythe HA, Yunus MB, et al. The American College of Rheumatology 1990 criteria for the classification of fibromyalgia. Report of the Multicenter Criteria Committee. *Arthritis Rheum*. 1990;33:160-172.

5   Gout

One of the most historically prominent rheumatic diseases (recognized by the ancient Greeks in the fifth century BC), gout should be thought of as a metabolic disease that has musculoskeletal consequences. The present term gout comes from the Latin, *gutta*, meaning "to drop." Therapy for gout dates to the middle ages when colchicine was introduced, and refinements of therapy have progressed to the point that, in a compliant patient, there are but rare situations where complete control of the disease should not occur.

Pathogenesis

Gout represents one of the best understood rheumatic disorders and is due to the phlogistic properties of monosodium urate crystals deposited in soft tissue. Uric acid is the end product of purine metabolism in man (Figure 5.1). Both dietary and *de novo* production account for endogenous purines. Regulation of purine production occurs predominantly through control of two enzymes, phosphoribosyl-pyrophosphate (PRPP) synthetase and amido-phosphoribosyltransferase (amido-PRT). Amido-PRT activity is enhanced in the presence of PRPP and inhibited by purine nucleotides. PRPP synthetase activity is also inhibited by purine nucleotides, but less so than amido-PRT. Increased activity of PRPP synthetase ultimately results in increases in production of uric acid.

The salvage pathway involving hypoxanthine-guanine phosphoribosyltransferase (HGPRT) is also important to note because of its clinical relevance. HGPRT catalyzes the conversion of hypoxanthine to

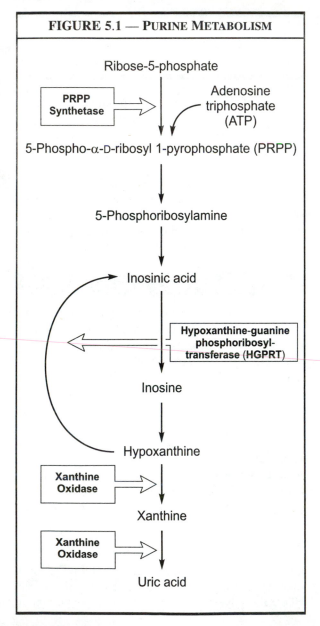

FIGURE 5.1 — PURINE METABOLISM

Ribose-5-phosphate

PRPP Synthetase

Adenosine triphosphate (ATP)

5-Phospho-α-D-ribosyl 1-pyrophosphate (PRPP)

5-Phosphoribosylamine

Inosinic acid

Hypoxanthine-guanine phosphoribosyl-transferase (HGPRT)

Inosine

Hypoxanthine

Xanthine Oxidase

Xanthine

Xanthine Oxidase

Uric acid

inosinic acid and hence purine salvage. The X-linked disorder, Lesch-Nyhan syndrome, is associated with absence of HGPRT activity and massive overproduction of uric acid.

The majority of the uric acid pool is produced from turnover of endogenous purines. Dietary purines account for the remaining minority of uric acid. Thus, only the most extreme diets are effective in decreasing serum concentrations of uric acid.

About two thirds of daily uric acid excretion is through the kidney, via a complicated renal handling mechanism. Nearly all serum uric acid is filtered through the glomerulus and the majority of this is reabsorbed in the proximal tubule. More distally, in the proximal tubule, there is secretion and again reabsorption. Overall, about 10% of the originally filtered load appears in the urine. The remainder of uric acid excretion is through the gastrointestinal (GI) tract, where it is subjected to the action of bacterial uricase, an enzyme not found in man.

The uric acid pool increases in men at puberty and in women at the menopause. The uric acid pool in men is about 1200 mg, twice that typically seen in women. Patients with gout invariably have an increased uric acid pool. Typically they have normal or increased renal excretion of uric acid. In comparison to individuals who are not hyperuricemic, most patients (over 90%) will have less uric acid appearing (when controlled for serum uric acid concentrations) in the urine than normouricemic controls. Additional factors may alter the production or renal handling of uric acid (Table 5.1). Increased cell turnover (eg, disorders such as the myelo- or lymphoproliferative disorders) increases production of uric acid. Similarly, factors which impair renal excretion, including glomerular dysfunction, or factors affecting tubular handling of uric acid (especially organic acids) increase levels of uric acid.

TABLE 5.1 — FACTORS ALTERING URIC ACID

Increased Urate Production
- Enhanced tissue turnover:
  - Hematological malignancies
  - Hemolysis
  - Psoriasis
  - Ethanol
  - Myositis
  - Tissue ischemia and necrosis
  - Trauma with crush injuries
- Drugs:
  - Ethanol
  - Chemotherapeutic agents
  - Nicotinic acid
  - Pyrazinamide

Decreased Renal Excretion
- Metabolic disorders and illnesses:
  - Dehydration
  - Lactic acidosis
  - Ketoacidosis
  - Lead intoxication
  - Bartter's syndrome
  - Renal failure
  - Fasting
- Drugs:
  - Ethanol
  - Diuretics
  - Salicylates
  - NSAIDs (variable effect)
  - Cyclosporine
  - Pyrazinamide

Abbreviation: NSAID, nonsteroidal anti-inflammatory drug.

Uric acid has a solubility of about 6.5 mg/dL in water. Concentrations greater than this represent supersaturated solutions and make precipitation of monosodium urate possible. Usually after many years of hyperuricemia, body stores of uric acid have increased to the point that adaptation to the excess is no longer possible, and clinically discernable disease results.

Crystals of monosodium urate free in the joint activate a number of inflammatory pathways. The crystals are coated with immunoglobin G (IgG), which activates complement. Similarly, the kallikrein system is activated. As a result, there is vasodilatation and influx of neutrophils. Phagocytosed uric acid crystals stimulate neutrophils to release prostaglandins and lysosomal enzymes and induce oxidant production. Further, neutrophils are unable to digest the phagocytosed urate crystal, which ultimately results in lysosomal rupture, cell death, and spillage of cellular contents extracellularly. Simultaneously, free uric acid crystals activate mononuclear cells and synoviocytes with the production of inflammatory cytokines, including interleukin (IL)-1 and tumor necrosis factor (TNF)-α, which account for some of the systemic symptoms seen particularly in recurrent attacks of gout.

Occurrence

Gout is a common disorder, particularly in men. Population surveys have indicated that about 5% or more of men are hyperuricemic. Hyperuricemia is more likely to occur in men and women who:

- Are overweight
- Have renal dysfunction
- Drink alcohol.

Overall, prevalence rates indicate that gout appears in about 1 out of every 500 individuals.

Clinical Presentation

Gout should be thought of as the end of a progression from asymptomatic hyperuricemia to clinical disease. Most patients found to have gout will have had elevated serum concentrations for a number of years. As noted above, this elevation may occur in men at puberty and in women at the menopause. Thus, it is not unusual to see men in their thirties or forties presenting with symptoms suggestive of gout, whereas women are often in their sixties or older.

Most patients will present with an acute attack involving one or (less likely) a few joints in the lower extremity. Often a history of self-limiting twinges involving a joint of the lower extremity that had been noticed in the weeks or months prior to the diagnostic episode can be elicited. A number of factors have been noted which appear to precipitate attacks of gout. Basically these are factors which alter serum concentrations of uric acid. Included would be:

- Alcohol binges
- Surgery
- Trauma
- Institution of diuretics
- Institution of uric acid-lowering agents.

The diagnostic attack generally occurs abruptly. Patients often note that they went to bed well and woke unable to walk because of pain. The involved joint often is red and swollen. Men typically present initially with involvement of the foot, and about half of the time with the first metatarsophalangeal (MTP). Interestingly, women may be more likely to have polyarticular attacks with involvement of the upper extremity. Other joints often involved early in the course of

60

the disease include the ankle, the midtarsals, the heel, the knee, and other sites such as the olecranon bursa. Involvement of the axial skeleton is not characteristic of gout.

A number of factors have been posited as reasons for involvement of the lower extremity. Uric acid solubility is temperature dependent and thus colder peripheral joints would be less likely to maintain its solubility. Further, hyaluronic acid, a major component of articular cartilage, increases the solubility of uric acid. In cultures where shoes are usually worn, osteoarthritis and its attendant loss of hyaluronic acid in the first MTP is common, thus limiting solubility of uric acid in the joint. Finally, it has been suggested that, with ambulation, the simple trauma causes fluid to enter the joint. At night, water is more rapidly absorbed from the joint than uric acid, increasing the concentration of uric acid, thus potentially causing its precipitation and triggering an attack.

The initial attack of gout usually resolves within several days to several weeks, despite the fact that crystals are still present in the joint. A number of changes in the joint may account for this observation. Crystals absorb apolipoprotein B, which makes the crystals less phlogistic. Further, crystals obtained later in the attack are smaller, which also has been shown to decrease their phlogistic properties. *Ex vivo*, exposure of monosodium urate crystals to oxygen radicals, does decrease crystal size. Lastly, during the acute response, apolipoprotein A1 is displaced from high-density lipoprotein, which may then inhibit neutrophil responsiveness.

Once the acute attack of gout has resolved, the patient enters into what is called the intercritical phase. This phase ends with the next attack of gout. The duration of the intercritical period is variable. It can last a few days or weeks and some patients may never have another attack of gout. To a large extent, the likelihood of having another attack is related to the serum concentration of uric acid. However, most patients will have a recurrence within the following 2 years.

The subsequent attacks of gout may be different, in that there is more likelihood to involve multiple joints and joints of the upper extremity. Additionally, the severity of the attack may be worse, with systemic features including high fever and chills, which may raise the consideration of sepsis or a septic joint.

In some patients who are left untreated, the intercritical periods will grow shorter or completely disappear, leaving the patient with chronic unremitting joint symptoms and progressive joint damage. This condition may be concordant with the appearance of tophi or accumulations of monosodium urate in the soft tissue. Tophi, which may have diagnostic importance, are found in a number of locations, including:

- Pinnae of the ears
- Fingers or toes
- Achilles tendon
- Olecranon bursa.

Laboratory Tests and Radiographs

Prior to the acute attack of gout or during the intercritical phase, laboratory tests will be normal apart from hyperuricemia. During an acute attack, acute phase proteins and white blood cell (WBC) counts are often elevated. Occasionally, a patient unequivocally has gout but has a normal serum uric acid. Synovial fluid is characteristically inflammatory, with an elevated WBC count. Most of the synovial fluid WBCs are neutrophils. Examination of the fluid will reveal negatively birefringent crystals (Figure 5.2). Even during the intercritical period, aspiration of previously involved joints will often disclose crystals, which may be helpful in making the diagnosis.

FIGURE 5.2 — URIC ACID CRYSTAL

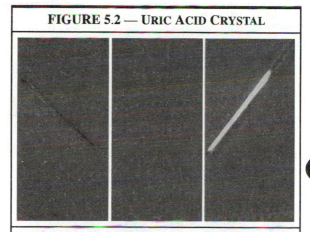

A polarized micrograph of a monosodium urate crystal. Note the long, needle-shaped crystals and bright birefringent pattern.

Courtesy of Arthritis Foundation.

Radiographs of involved joints early in the course show only nonspecific changes such as soft-tissue swelling. As the disease progresses, erosions occur which characteristically are punched-out lesions with a sclerotic margin (Figure 5.3). Often these erosions will appear off the margin of the joint, which helps to differentiate them from the erosions of rheumatoid arthritis. Additionally, there tend to be no signs of periarticular osteoporosis. Intraosseus or soft tissue tophi may be apparent on radiographs.

Diagnosis

Gout is most often considered in a patient who presents with either a mono- or oligoarthritis involving the lower extremity (Table 5.2). As noted above, patients with recurrent attacks or older women are less likely to have such a characteristic presentation. Once considered, the diagnosis is most readily made by as-

**FIGURE 5.3 — RADIOGRAPH
OF GOUT IN HAND**

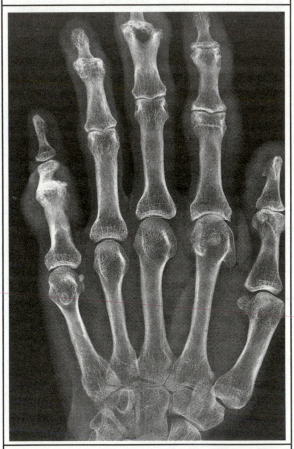

Radiograph of the hand from a patient with gout. Note
the relative absence of periarticular osteopenia. Erosions
tend to be "punched out" with sclerotic borders and tend
to occur in areas distinct from the cartilage pannus junction seen in rheumatoid arthritis. Note the soft tissue den-
sity particularly apparent around the fifth digit which represents accumulation of monosodium urate.

TABLE 5.2 — DIFFERENTIAL DIAGNOSIS OF GOUT

- Abrupt onset
- Oligoarthritis
- Lower-extremity involvement
- Presence of tophi

pirating the involved joint and demonstrating intracellular crystals compatible with monosodium urate. In most situations, this is accomplished by observing fresh fluid under the polarized microscope. Refrigerating synovial fluid may precipitate uric acid crystals and confuse the diagnosis. Monosodium urate crystals are distinctive for their needle shape and negatively birefringent optical characteristics (Figure 5.2).

Simply demonstrating that a patient with arthritis has hyperuricemia is not adequate to diagnose gout. Patients with renal failure often have dramatically elevated serum uric acid concentrations but, apart from those with polycystic kidney disease, may not develop symptoms of gouty arthritis. A number of disorders, including pseudogout, osteoarthritis, stress fractures, and even septic arthritis, may simulate this picture. Nonetheless, a patient with hyperuricemia who develops a monoarthritis and responds dramatically to colchicine often is presumed to have gout.

Management

There is no evidence that treating a patient with asymptomatic hyperuricemia is useful; it does expose the patient to the risk and expense of therapy. Treatment of the patient with gout can be divided into strategies directed toward:

- Therapy of acute attacks
- Uric acid-lowering therapy
- Prophylactic therapy.

■ Therapy of Acute Attacks

The response to therapy of an acute attack of gout is dependent upon the rapidity with which therapy is instituted. Well-developed attacks may take several days to respond, while premonitory twinges may respond in minutes or hours.

Nonsteroidal Anti-inflammatory Drugs

Traditionally, the acute attack of gout has been treated with either nonsteroidal anti-inflammatory drugs (NSAIDs) or colchicine. If NSAIDs are used, it is important to obtain anti-inflammatory levels of these medications. Thus, for NSAIDs with long half-lives, traditional dosing regimens are generally slow in reaching full anti-inflammatory levels. In contrast, drugs with short half-lives, such as ibuprofen or indomethacin, achieve full anti-inflammatory doses rapidly. As always, care must be taken administering these drugs to patients with a history of acid peptic disease or who have the potential for renal dysfunction when cyclooxygenase activity is blocked.

Colchicine

Colchicine is an alternative and effective therapy for acute gout. A number of dosing regimens have been recommended over the years. One regimen recommends 0.6 mg of colchicine every hour until side effects intervene or the acute attack has resolved. GI side effects usually occur prior to a symptomatic response. Alternatively, colchicine can be administered intravenously. Caution must be exercised with this route of administration as it is a vesicant, and extravasation can cause tissue necrosis. Nonetheless, care must be taken when using colchicine in patients who have underlying renal or hepatic disease, where its accumulation may result in marrow toxicity.

Corticosteroids

Frequently, coexisting medical conditions, namely transplants or renal dysfunction, preclude the use of either NSAIDs or colchicine. In those situations, corticosteroids will control the process until other methods can be implemented. If a single joint is involved, intra-articular steroids may be adequate to control the process. If several joints are active, either steroids or intramuscular adrenocorticotropic hormone (ACTH) are effective in controlling the disease. Prednisone or equivalent in doses of 20 to 40 mg is usually quite effective. After several days, the dose can be quickly tapered. Alternatively, ACTH given as about 40 U is effective, but patients may require additional therapy within a few days.

■ Uric Acid-Lowering Therapy

Once the acute attack has resolved, a decision usually needs to be made regarding uric acid-lowering agents. Since many patients will go for long periods of time without another attack, one approach would be to simply wait and see. During this time, decrease or remove contributing factors, such as:

- Obesity
- Alcohol abuse
- Medications that elevate uric acid.

Alternatively, uric acid-lowering therapy may be instituted in the patient who has multiple recurrent attacks or whose initial attack was severe.

It is often recommended that a 24-hour urine collection for uric acid be performed before beginning uric acid-lowering therapy. This is cumbersome and, in many situations, nearly impossible. Recommendations for this collection include 5 days of a purine-free isocaloric diet, followed by two 24-hour collections. This must be performed while the patient is off medications, which may interfere with the renal excretion of uric acid, and is only meaningful in a patient who has normal renal function. Since most patients (about 90%) will be relative underexcretors of uric acid, uricosuric agents can often be used without determining 24-hour urinary uric acid excretion.

Uricosuric Agents

Uricosuric agents decrease the concentration of uric acid in the blood by increasing the renal excretion of this molecule. Candidates for these medications include patients who:
- Are underexcretors
- Have normal renal function
- Have not had renal calculi.

During institution of these medications, renal excretion of uric acid increases, which may supersaturate the urine and predispose for the production of renal calculi. Adequate hydration, particularly in hot climates, is important to limit this risk. Once the body stores and blood levels of uric acid have been decreased, renal excretion of uric acid returns to the baseline provided that renal function has remained stable and the uricosuric agent is continued. Probenecid and sulfinpyrazone are available in the United States, and recommended dosing regimens are listed in Table 5.3. Doses of each agent are titrated up until serum concentrations of uric acid are < 6 mg/dL. Lack of response to uricosuric agents is due to:
- Insufficient renal function
- Poor compliance
- Compounds (such as salicylates) which may interfere with their action
- Extreme elevation of uric acid.

Most patients are tolerant of these drugs. Risks of renal calculi are diminished by gradually increasing the
68

TABLE 5.3 — URICOSURICS		
Drug	**Initial Dose**	**Maximum Dose (Total Daily)**
Probenecid	250 mg bid	3000 mg bid or tid
Sulfinpyrazone	50 mg bid	600 mg bid or tid

dose and hydration. Other side effects include skin rashes and, rarely, marrow toxicity. Sulfinpyrazone also has antiplatelet activity which may have beneficial effects.

Allopurinol

Patients who are candidates for uric acid-lowering therapy may also be treated with agents that interfere with the production of uric acid. These agents are particularly indicated in patients with gout who:

- Are intolerant of uricosurics
- Have found uricosurics ineffective
- Have renal insufficiency
- Have renal calculi
- Have tophaceous gout.

The most frequently used agent is allopurinol. It is an analog of hypoxanthine and works as an inhibitor of xanthine oxidase. Thus, both the conversion of hypoxanthine to xanthine and xanthine to uric acid is inhibited. Most patients tolerate allopurinol well. The most common side effect is a mild skin rash, but exfoliating disorders have been reported. A more serious side effect, termed allopurinol hypersensitivity syndrome, is manifested by:

- A diffuse vasculitic rash
- Eosinophilia
- Hepatic dysfunction with elevated liver enzymes
- Occasionally death.

Many of these descriptions of allopurinol hypersensitivity have been in older patients with renal dysfunction who were started on 300 mg/d or more. Thus, it has been recommended that in older patients or those with renal dysfunction, therapy should be initiated with lower doses, ie, 100 mg/d and slowly titrated up. In general, doses of allopurinol can be increased by about 100 mg/d every 3 weeks with the intention of decreasing serum levels to < 6 mg/dL. This goal can be reached in most patients with doses of about 300 mg/d, but occasionally patients need doses as high as 800 mg or more. Patients who are intolerant of allopurinol may be treated with oxypurinol. This agent is poorly absorbed from the GI tract and is not readily available in the United States.

■ **Prophylactic Agents**

Regardless of the therapy used to lower serum levels of uric acid, acute attacks of gout may be precipitated by initiation of therapy. It is generally recommended that prophylactic agents be used during this phase of therapy. Colchicine administered 2 to 3 times a day or NSAIDs are equally effective. Once the level of uric acid has decreased, these agents can usually be discontinued.

SUGGESTED READING

Campion EW, Glynn RJ, DeLabry LO. Asymptomatic hyperuricemia. Risks and conseqeunces in the Normative Aging Study. *Am J Med*. 1987;82:421-426.

Gutman AB. The past four decades of progress in the knowledge of gout, with an assessment of the present status. *Arthritis Rheum*. 1973;16:431-445.

Hall AP, Barry PE, Dawber TR, McNamara PM. Epidemiology of gout and hyperuricemia. A long-term population study. *Am J Med*. 1967;42:27-37.

Puig JG, Michán AD, Jiménez ML, et al. Female gout. Clinical spectrum and uric acid metabolism. *Arch Intern Med*. 1991;151: 726-732.

Wallace SL, Robinson H, Masi AT, Decker JL, McCarty DJ, Yü T. Preliminary criteria for the classification of the acute arthritis of primary gout. *Arthritis Rheum*. 1977;20:895-900.

5

6

Juvenile Chronic Arthritis

Juvenile chronic arthritis (JCA) is the term presently used to describe several childhood clinical syndromes where arthritis is prominent. By definition, those with JCA are under 16 years of age, but the presentation and course include:

- Oligoarthritis
- Polyarthritis
- Domination by systemic features of the disease.

Pathogenesis

As with many inflammatory rheumatic diseases, there appears to be at least a genetic predisposition to the development of JCA. However, many of the putative genetic risk factors have not been fully elucidated or confirmed. This is in part due to the fact that the form of arthritis that a patient with JCA has may evolve. Patients may have oligoarticular disease at the onset, but later progress to the polyarticular form, thus confusing classification. Nonetheless, patients who have systemic disease may have the human leukocyte antigen (HLA)-DR4 antigen more often, whereas those who have HLA-DR8 and HLA-DR5 may have a more benign course.

Occurrence

The prevalence of JCA is about one tenth that of adult rheumatoid arthritis, thus, less than one out of a thousand children will have one of the clinical presentations of the disease. A pauciarticular presentation is the most common, seen in about half of children with JCA. A polyarticular presentation is slightly less common, and a systemic onset is seen in about 10% of cases. Those with systemic onset are as likely to be boys as girls, but the other two presentations tend to occur more often in girls.

Clinical Features

■ Pauciarticular Onset

Pauciarticular presentation is most often seen in very young girls (often less that 4 years of age) and involves four or fewer joints (the knee most commonly). Anterior uveitis is frequently seen in this group, and most will not report eye symptoms before vision is impaired.

Children of this age may not be able to articulate their joint problems, but may instead simply refuse to use the joint. For example, those with involvement of the knee or hip may refuse to walk. As might be expected, of the three presentations of JCA, those with pauciarticular disease have the best prognosis. Less than half will have symptoms that last over 10 years, and fewer will develop erosions.

■ Polyarticular Onset

Polyarticular presentation is generally seen in older girls (typically over 7 or 8 years of age) and involves five or more joints. Patients may be initially thought to have pauciarticular disease. Systemic symptoms may be seen, such as:

- Fatigue
- Morning stiffness
- Low-grade fever.

Uveitis is typically seen with this disease, and eye examinations are an important part of management.

In those who are seronegative for rheumatoid factor, the arthritis is generally symmetrical and frequently involves the small joints of the hands and feet. Knee involvement is also common and is frequently associated with disability. Temporomandibular joint involvement may interfere with eating and often leads to a characteristic micrognathia.

Approximately 50% of these children will develop erosive disease. A polyarticular presentation is also seen in older girls, particularly young teenagers, who are seropositive for rheumatoid factor. Their presentation may be indistinguishable from that seen in adult rheumatoid arthritis.

■ Systemic Onset

Systemic onset is the least common form of JCA, but the presentation is frequently the most impressive and includes:

- Onset under 6 or 7 years of age
- May present with spiking fevers usually along with the arthritis, but the fever may antedate other features of the disease by weeks or months
- Affects boys and girls equally
- Variable in severity and number of joints involved
- May be a symmetrical polyarthritis with the hands usually involved
- Uveitis is unusual with systemic presentation.

Perhaps most characteristic of the extra-articular features is the skin rash of systemic onset JCA. Salmon colored, this evanescent eruption is often seen over joints, palms or soles (Figure 6.1). It may be asymptomatic or slightly pruritic and often appears with heat or fever. Other children with systemic JCA may develop hepatosplenomegaly, lymphadenopathy, vasculitis, pericarditis with effusions and, less often, pulmonary hypertension.

FIGURE 6.1 — RASH OF
JUVENILE CHRONIC ARTHRITIS

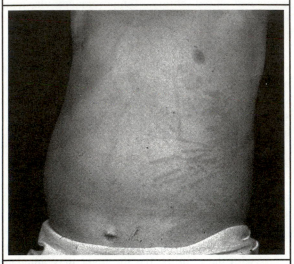

The rash of juvenile chronic arthritis is often evanescent. This blanching rash may be seen during times of fever or stress.

Courtesy of Arthritis Foundation.

Laboratory Tests and Radiographs

There are no laboratory tests specific for JCA. Older children with polyarticular onset, as noted above, may be positive for rheumatoid factor. Antinuclear antibodies (ANA) are seen:

- Frequently in children with a pauciarticular presentation
- In about half of those with polyarticular disease
- In about 10% of those with systemic onset.

The presence of ANA, particularly in those with pauciarticular onset, is strongly linked to the development of uveitis.

Abnormalities in other laboratory tests reflect systemic inflammation. Erythrocyte sedimentation rates and C-reactive protein are elevated, as are platelet and often white blood cell (WBC) counts. Children may have anemia of chronic disease. Synovial fluids generally are inflammatory in nature, with elevated WBC counts, most of which are neutrophils.

Radiographs may be helpful in some patients with JCA. Erosions or cartilage loss may be difficult to visualize with plain radiographs in the not-fully-mature joint. Osteopenia or soft-tissue swelling may be the only clues early in the disease. Certainly some may develop advanced changes with erosions and deformity, but in those situations the diagnosis is rarely in doubt. Chronic inflammation may increase growth at the joint leading to bony overgrowth. Alternatively, growth plates may be closed prematurely leading to shortening of the bone.

Diagnosis

In many patients, the initial history and examination can lead to the correct diagnosis of JCA. Criteria have been developed which may be helpful (Table 6.1). Depending upon the pattern of onset, a number of other disorders should be considered such as:

- Infectious arthritis in those who have a pauci-articular onset
- Joint pain associated with human immunodeficiency virus (HIV) infection
- Lyme disease (may be polyarticular)
- The seronegative spondyloarthropathies, particularly juvenile ankylosing spondylitis, may be a consideration when a child presents with arthritis and axial disease or with other extra-articular features such as psoriasis

TABLE 6.1 — GENERAL CRITERIA FOR JUVENILE RHEUMATOID ARTHRITIS

Persistent arthritis of one or more joints for at least 6 weeks is sufficient for diagnosis if conditions listed have been eliminated.

Other Rheumatic Diseases
- Rheumatic fever
- Systemic lupus erythematosus
- Ankylosing spondylitis
- Polymyositis and dermatomyositis
- Vasculitis:
  - Anaphylactoid purpura (Henoch-Schönlein)
  - Polyarteritis
  - Serum sickness and other allergic reactions
  - Mucocutaneous lymph node syndrome: infantile polyarteritis
  - Other causes of arthritis
- Scleroderma
- Psoriatic arthritis
- Reiter's syndrome
- Sjögren's syndrome
- Mixed connective tissue disease
- Behçet's syndrome

Infectious Arthritis
- Bacterial arthritis, including tuberculosis
- Viral, fungal, and mycoplasmal arthritides
- Nonbacterial arthritis associated with bacterial infections
- Other causes of arthritis

Inflammatory Bowel Disease

Neoplastic Diseases, Including Leukemia

Nonrheumatic Conditions of Bones and Joints
- Osteochondritis
- Toxic synovitis of the hip
- Slipped capital femoral epiphyses
- Trauma:
  - Battered child syndrome
  - Fractures

Continued

> – Joint, ligamentous, and muscular injuries
> – Congenital indifference to pain
> – Acute chondrolysis
> • Chondromalacia of the patella
> • Congenital anomalies and genetically determined abnormalities of the musculoskeletal system, including inborn errors of metabolism

Brewer EJ Jr, et al. *Arthritis Rheum.* 1977;20(suppl 2):195-199.

- Local disorders (ie, bursitis)
- Hip pain due to slipped capital femoral epiphyses or Legg-Calvé-Perthes disease
- Knee pain due to chondromalacia patella
- Diffuse joint pain simply due to:
  - Growing pains
  - Leukemic infiltration or other malignancies
  - Sickle cell disease
  - Inherited abnormalities of connective tissues.

Management

The goal of treatment of the child with JCA is not only directed toward the articular disease, but also to limit the psychosocial damage related to a chronic illness. In many situations, this may require a multi-faceted team approach, including:

- Teachers
- Counselors
- Social workers
- Parents
- Therapists
- Other health-care providers.

■ Nonpharmacological Therapy

Even when focusing on the articular disease, a number of nonpharmacological measures are useful. Passive stretching and exercise to maintain range of motion and muscle strength are helpful. Splints may be useful for limiting pain and maintaining positioning in those with inflamed joints or deformity. In those with flexion contractures, serial casting may return joint motion toward normal. Other devices help with leg length discrepancies or ankle instability.

■ Pharmacological Therapy
Nonsteroidal Anti-inflammatory Drugs

Pharmacological therapy is usually initiated with a nonsteroidal anti-inflammatory drug (NSAID) (Table 6.2). Most children will respond to these agents; lack of response of some sort should raise the question of compliance or toxicity. Pragmatic considerations, such as cost or frequency of dosing, usually guide NSAID choice since there is no data demonstrating superiority of one agent above the rest.

Aspirin has a long history of efficacy at anti-inflammatory doses in JCA, but it does have a narrow therapeutic index. Dosing can be guided by blood drug levels and the reporting of tinnitus, which is often the first sign of toxicity. However, very young children may not be able to report that they are experiencing this symptom. There is no evidence that combining NSAIDs is useful and this practice may lead to increased adverse events. Thus, it would seem prudent to caution against over-the-counter use of NSAIDs, when a prescription is provided. Those whose pain symptoms are not adequately controlled with an NSAID can be treated with acetaminophen.

Corticosteroids

Corticosteroid use is often an important component of the pharmacological therapy of JCA. In children with systemic disease, their use may be life-saving. Doses of 1 to 2 mg/kg/d are often needed, and the dose may need to be divided. Once symptoms are controlled, the dose should be tapered. Chil-

TABLE 6.2 — NONSTEROIDAL ANTI-INFLAMMATORY DRUGS USED FOR JUVENILE RHEUMATOID ARTHRITIS

Generic Name	Trade Name	Manufacturer	Delivery Method	Recommended Dosage
Aspirin	Ecotrin	SmithKline Beecham	Tablets	4000 mg/d in divided doses, ie, up to 650 mg q4h or 1000 mg q6h
Ibuprofen	Motrin	McNeil	Suspension Oral Drops Chewable Tablets Caplets	30 to 40 mg/kg/d in divided doses (tid or qid)
Naproxen	Naprosyn	Roche	Suspension	10 mg/kg/d in divided doses (bid)
Tolmetin sodium	Tolectin	Ortho-McNeil	Tablets Capsules	20 mg/kg/d in divided doses (tid or qid)

Physicians' Desk Reference. 53rd ed. Montvale, NJ: Medical Economics Company, Inc; 1999.

6

dren with pauci- or polyarticular disease may benefit from low doses of corticosteroids. Typically about 0.1 mg/kg/d administered in the morning can limit pain, swelling and stiffness. Patients with pauciarticular JCA or in those who have only a few active joints, may alternatively benefit from intra-articular corticosteroids. In addition to other effects, long-term, high-dose corticosteroids lead to growth suppression. Topical steroids are usually needed to control uveitis, if present; rarely, systemic steroids may be necessary.

Slow-Acting Antirheumatic Drugs

Only about one third of children will have their articular disease controlled with NSAIDs alone; the remainder are candidates for slow-acting antirheumatic drugs (SAARDs). Most rheumatologists prefer methotrexate over other SAARDs as the initial therapy for JCA. Response is dose dependent and the minimal, effective dose appears to be 10 mg/m^2 given weekly. Toxicity is also dose dependent, with mucositis and nausea being the more common side effects. Treatment with folic acid may diminish side effects.

Parenteral gold, prior to being displaced by methotrexate, had been the leading SAARD for JCA. After administering test doses, children are given 1/mg/kg/wk for about 20 weeks. Subsequent gold therapy is guided by response and toxicity. About 50% to 65% will respond, but the response is often incomplete. Common toxicities are:
- Rash
- Proteinuria
- Cytopenias.

The injectable, soluble TNF-α receptor, etanercept (Enbrel), has been shown to be effective in JRA and provides an alternative therapy to those children who have failed conventional therapies.

Other Agents

Other agents that have achieved at least anecdotal success as therapies for JCA include hydroxychloroquine, penicillamine, and oral gold, but controlled studies failed to indicate benefit above placebo. Sulfasalazine also has been used successfully in uncontrolled studies. A number of other agents, including azathioprine, cyclosporin A, and intravenous immunoglobulin G (IgG), have been tried in an attempt to manage resistant disease.

■ Surgery

Surgical intervention may be important in selected children with JCA. Soft-tissue releases can improve range of motion, which may be particularly important in the hip or knee. Postoperative physical therapy is critical if motion is to be maintained. Children who have developed leg length discrepancies (eg, increased growth of the limb because of asymmetrical involvement of a knee where the growth plate has fused) may benefit from timed fusion on the growth plate on the other knee. In general, joint replacements are reserved until the child is an older adult because of the limited duration of the prosthesis.

6

SUGGESTED READING

Arnett FC. Revised criteria for the classification of rheumatoid arthritis. *Bull Rheum Dis*. 1989;38:1-6.

Brewer EL Jr, Bass J, Baum J, et al. Current proposed revision of JRA Criteria. JRA Criteria Subcommittee of the Diagnostic and Therapeutic Criteria Committee of the American Rheumatism Section of The Arthritis Foundation. *Arthritis Rheum*. 1977;20(suppl 2):195-199.

Gäre BA, Fasth A. The natural history of juvenile chronic arthritis: a population based cohort study. II. Outcome. *J Rheumatol*. 1995;22:308-319.

Kremer JM, Alarcón GS, Lightfoot RW Jr, et al. Methotrexate for rheumatoid arthritis. Suggested guidelines for monitoring liver toxicity. American College of Rheumatology. *Arthritis Rheum*. 1994;37:316-328.

Towner S, Michet CJ Jr, O'Fallon WM, Nelson AM. The epidemiology of juvenile arthritis in Rochester, Minnesota, 1960-1979. *Arthritis Rheum*. 1983;26:1208-1213.

Yancey C, Gross R. Guidelines for opthalmologic examinaiton in children with juvenile rheumatoid arthritis. *Pediatrics*. 1993;92: 295-296.

7 Low Back Pain

Nearly every person will experience an episode of low back pain; many will be at least transiently disabling. A whole host of therapies and the seemingly endless list of diagnostic tests have been applied to the problem, at times with confusion and, all too often, without improving the patient's problem. For most individuals, a conservative approach to diagnosis and therapy is more likely to be helpful.

7

Pathogenesis

After one walks upright for even a short span of years, the lumbar spine shows evidence of degenerative changes. The lumbar discs, composed of a central elastic nucleus pulposus and surrounding annulus fibrosis, are thinned and the nucleus pulposus may protrude through the annulus. Occasionally, the herniated disc material may impinge upon a nerve root. Subjacent vertebral bodies are thickened and osteophytes may form. Similar changes are frequently seen in the articular facet joints.

The closer one looks at the lumbar spine, the more likely one is to find abnormalities, even in those with no history of back pain. Despite these observations, pinpointing the site of pain in an individual with low back pain is often not feasible.

Occurrence

Back pain is common. Symptoms usually begin in adolescence or early adulthood and may plague individuals for the rest of their lives. Next to upper respiratory infections, it is the leading cause of visits to primary-care physicians. Surveys have indicated that over 80% of adults recall an episode of low back pain; 40% recall the episode as disabling. Overall, men are seen with low back pain slightly more often than women (Table 7.1).

TABLE 7.1 — RISK FACTORS FOR NONDEGENERATIVE LOW BACK PAIN

- Older age
- Location of pain:
  - Upper lumbar
  - Lower thoracic spine
- Recent spinal manipulation
- Intravenous drug use
- History of systemic symptoms:
  - Fever
  - Weight loss

Clinical Presentation

Patients seeking medical care for low back pain frequently have had several previous, self-limiting episodes of pain. In many situations, the precipitating event is trivial or not ascertainable. Discomfort is vaguely localized and may include radiation to the buttock or lateral leg. In most situations, the specific source of the pain is elusive, but has been variably attributed to:

- Degenerative changes in the vertebral discs or facet joints
- Instability due to spondylolisthesis
- Paraspinous muscle spasm.

Unfortunately, radiographs and other imaging techniques only rarely define the responsible structure in those with nonspecific back pain.

In those with nerve-root entrapment and pain, the most commonly implicated roots are those between L4 and L5 or L5 and S1. Patients may note that maneuvers which increase intraspinal pressure, such as coughing or the Valsalva maneuver, increase pain. Similarly, sitting or standing may exacerbate symptoms.

In general, the L4 nerve provides sensation to the posterolateral thigh, the anterior knee, and medial leg. L5's innervation is more lateral and usually includes the great toe. However, localization of the entrapped nerve root by sensory examination alone is often incorrect.

Straight leg is often positive in those with entrapped nerve roots, particularly in younger individuals, but hip or pelvic disease or tight hamstrings may limit application of this test. Evidence of muscle weakness may be of further help in defining an entrapped nerve root. Heel walking tests the L5 innervated ankle dorsiflexors, whereas the plantar flexors, tested by toe walking, are predominantly innervated by S1. Reflex abnormalities may also be helpful, as a decreased hamstring reflex with a normal ankle jerk suggests an L5 lesion. It should be remembered that in older individuals or those with disorders such as diabetes, reflex abnormalities are common.

Apart from herniated discs, there are a number of other structures that may cause compressive symptoms and are generally considered under the heading of spinal stenosis. Congenitally small vertebral columns, postoperative fibrosis, hypertrophic ligamentum flavum, and degenerative changes with compressive osteophytes have all been cited as causes of spinal stenosis. Most individuals thought to have back pain due to spinal stenosis are older and often relate a long history of low back pain. Leg pain with walking, with a normal vascular examination, is suggestive. Increasing pain with walking downhill and the increased lumbar lordosis is another clue.

Individuals with osteoporosis may develop compression fractures. Usually they are acute in onset and the pain excruciating in severity, but frequently resolve in 4 to 6 weeks. Multiparous, postmenopausal women are at greatest risk. Steroid use, lack of exercise, alcohol and cigarette abuse are other risk factors for osteoporosis.

Infections and tumors are often cited as reasons for further evaluation of a patient with backache, but these are truly unusual causes of back pain. Certain symptoms, including nocturnal pain while recumbent, localized tenderness over a spinous process, fever or other unexplained systemic symptoms, and upper lumbar and lower thoracic pain suggest that other causes may be operative. Osteomyelitis of the vertebral column is usually secondary to hematogenous spread and typically involves at least two vertebral bodies and the intervening disc. Intravenous drug use and endocarditis are risk factors. Those with intra-abdominal catastrophes and who have had spinal instrumentation which may have resulted in seeding of the vertebral bodies are other risk factors.

Epidural abscesses are equally due to spread from an adjacent vertebrae, local infection, or hematogenous spread. Back pain is often localized, but systemic symptoms may be absent. Pain is progressive and is often associated with signs of meningeal irritation. Once the abscess reaches a sufficient size, compressive symptoms may predominate.

Laboratory Tests and Radiographs

There are no tests or specific imaging procedures which can be cited as necessary or uniformly useful in evaluating the patient with low back pain. In most situations, none are needed. Indeed, a quixotic search using the latest technology is not only expensive and potentially harmful, but fortifies the patient's perspective that s/he is indeed sick. Some physicians obtain an erythrocyte sedimentation rate or complete blood count to help differentiate mechanical problems from systemic disorders.

Imaging procedures are of no specific help in managing the patient with routine backache. Nearly all adults will have degenerative changes on plain radiographs of the lumbosacral spine. Compression fractures may be visualized, but it is unusual to be able to ascertain their duration. Rapid dissolution of the intervertebral disc may suggest an infectious process. Replacement of the vertebral body may be seen in a patient with an abscess or metastatic disease.

If neurological symptoms prevail, magnetic resonance imaging may demonstrate a nerve root or cord impingement. Demonstration of bulging discs is common enough to be considered an essentially normal finding.

Diagnosis

In most cases of low back pain, the diagnosis can be made based on the history and physical examination alone. Often useful in the examination is observation as the patient stands and walks. Ankle dorsi and plantar flexors can be tested with heel and toe walking. In the sitting position, reflexes can be tested, quadriceps bulk can be determined and a sitting, straight-leg raising performed. With the patient supine, a hip, abdominal and vascular examination can be performed.

A more detailed evaluation may be prompted by:
- Historical findings or progressive unremitting pain
- Development of neurological deficits
- Unexplained systemic symptoms.

However, as noted above, physicians should be cautious regarding the unnecessary use of diagnostic tests. Development of demonstrable neurological deficits usually prompts the ordering of imaging procedures to determine the site.

Management

In most situations, back pain resolves in a matter of days to weeks. About 75% of patients will have resolution within a month and over 90% by 3 months. Studies evaluating the role of bed rest have not demonstrated that it in any way hastens resolution of back pain. Indeed, prolonged bed rest promotes deconditioning and rewards a "sick role."

Patients with acute low back pain are often treated with analgesics, including:

- Acetaminophen
- Nonsteroidal anti-inflammatory drugs (NSAIDs)
- Tramadol
- Narcotics.

Long-term therapy with acetaminophen is safest and not associated with the gastrointestinal and renal side effects seen with NSAIDs. Careful thought should be given prior to prescribing narcotic analgesics for more than a brief duration.

Much of the therapy likely to be effective in limiting recurrence of back pain is the responsibility of the patient. Weight control, proper posture and lifting techniques, and exercise are likely to be effective, and they are not invasive or costly. Exercises such as partial situps and leg lifts may be useful when coupled with stretching exercises (Figure 7.1). A number of modalities, such as ultrasound and transcutaneous nerve stimulators, have been offered as therapies, but are difficult to recommend as being better than placebo.

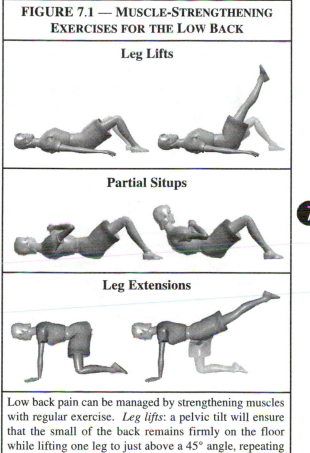

FIGURE 7.1 — MUSCLE-STRENGTHENING EXERCISES FOR THE LOW BACK

Leg Lifts

Partial Situps

Leg Extensions

Low back pain can be managed by strengthening muscles with regular exercise. *Leg lifts*: a pelvic tilt will ensure that the small of the back remains firmly on the floor while lifting one leg to just above a 45° angle, repeating for each side. Do not lock the knee. *Partial situps*: keeping the small of the back pressed firmly to the floor as in the leg lifts, duck the chin slightly into the chest and curl the upper torso upward just until the small of the back begins to lift. *Leg extensions*: on hands and knees, hold the abdominals in firmly and keep the back flat and straight; lift one leg just above horizontal to the floor, keeping knee relaxed. Repeat for each side.

Surgery is rarely indicated for management of routine low back pain. Even when neurological deficits are present and have been demonstrated to be associated with nerve-root entrapment, signs and symptoms often respond without surgical therapy. There is no convincing evidence that, over the long term, surgical intervention improves outcome in an unselected patient group with backache. Even in carefully selected patients, surgical intervention may not be effective more than half of the time. The "last resort" should not be an indication for surgical intervention, but instead point to progressive or unremitting neurological deficits.

SUGGESTED READING

Blackburn WD Jr, Alarcon GS, Ball GV. Evaluation of patients with back pain of suspected inflammatory nature. *Am J Med*. 1988;85:766-770.

Deyo RA, Tsui-Wu YJ. Descriptive epidemiology of low-back pain and its related medical care in the United States. *Spine*. 1987;12:264-268.

Hadler NM. Regional back pain. *N Engl J Med*. 1986;315: 1090-1092. Editorial.

Liang M, Komaroff AL. Roentgenograms in primary care patients with acute low back pain. *Arch Intern Med*. 1982;142:1108-1112.

8   Lyme Disease

The unfolding story of Lyme disease is a true representation of the ideal interaction between clinicians and basic biomedical researchers. An initial cluster of children with an inflammatory arthritis were seen in Lyme, Connecticut, leading to the recognition of Lyme disease as a syndrome in 1975. From that astute initial clinical observation, the clinical spectrum has been mapped, the cause determined, therapies devised, and prevention strategies formulated.

Pathogenesis

Initial studies determined that Lyme disease was linked to the bite of several small ticks. In the United States, most cases have been attributed to bites of the deer tick, *Ixodes scapularis*; in Europe, it has been principally linked to the sheep tick, *Ixodes ricinus*. Other ticks, notably the *Ixodes pacificus* and *Amblyomma americanum*, have been shown to harbor the etiologic agent responsible for Lyme disease.

These hard-body ticks are found in the United States predominantly in the northeast, midwest, and west, and are most active in the late spring and summer. Typically, they have a 2-year lifespan, composed of larva, nymph, and adult stages.

In 1982, the causative organism responsible for Lyme disease was isolated from an *Ixodes* tick. From culture and serological evidence, it has been firmly established that the spirochete *Borrelia burgdorferi* is the causative organism.

The spirochete is injected into the skin at the site of the tick bite. After a period of latency, lasting approximately 1 month, the organism migrates from the bite site and causes the characteristic annular rash. During this time, there may be dissemination to other sites, notably the joints, central nervous system (CNS), and heart.

Although some symptoms are clearly due to infection, there is evidence to suggest that some of the clinical manifestations occur even when the organism is not detectable. This has led to hypotheses, such as molecular mimicry, that are typically invoked to explain symptoms when an organism is not present.

Occurrence

Lyme disease is a seasonal disorder. Most commonly, initial manifestations occur in the summer and early fall, times concordant with the activity of the tick and likelihood of individuals being exposed to ticks. Most individuals with Lyme disease are children and young and middle-aged adults.

The number of individuals with Lyme disease is not fully known. It is a reportable disorder, but some patients may have Lyme disease and escape detection, whereas others may have serological evidence of exposure and be asymptomatic or have unrelated clinical symptoms. Nonetheless, approximately 10,000 new cases of Lyme disease are reported annually in the United States.

Clinical Features

As noted above, clinical manifestations are delayed after inoculation of the spirochete for as long as a month. The clinical hallmark of the disease is the rash, erythema migrans. Generally this begins as a small erythematous macule or papule which gradually enlarges and then may fade, even untreated, over a period of several weeks. As the lesion enlarges, the front is warm, erythematous, and usually nonpalpable. There may be central clearing, but also induration or necrosis. Secondary lesions may occur during this time, which represent dissemination of the organism, but these lesions usually are smaller than the primary lesion. Perhaps because of the relative lack of temporal contiguity between the tick bite and onset of symptoms, only about one third of patients will recall a tick bite at the site of the initial lesion.

Before or during the onset of erythema migrans, constitutional symptoms usually develop. Fatigue, malaise, fever, headaches, and arthralgias are often noted, and may be noted even without the rash, existing for months after the rash resolves.

Many patients will have this relatively self-limited illness, but a minority will proceed to develop other complications of Lyme disease. Arthritis is probably the most common sign of Lyme disease and likely develops in over 50% of symptomatic patients. Reports of intermittent myalgias and arthralgias for weeks or months prior to the development of physical signs indicative of arthritis are common. Although any joint may be involved, most commonly affected are the large joints, particularly the knee. Attacks of arthritis are usually sudden in onset and associated with fatigue and malaise. Effusions may be large and generally will resolve in several weeks, but recurrences are common. After months or several years, the frequency attacks of arthritis wanes. In a definite minority of patients, a proliferative synovitis develops, which is histologically reminiscent of rheumatoid arthritis. In these patients, there is an association with the class II human leukocyte antigen DR4 and the development of a humoral response to certain *B burgdorferi* surface proteins.

Neurological involvement may occur in the first several months of the disease. Headaches and signs of meningeal irritation and cognitive dysfunction are common neurological symptoms, as is evidence of peripheral nerve dysfunction, particularly of the cranial nerves and the facial nerve. These acute neurological symptoms usually resolve, but may take several months to do so.

Cardiac involvement, less common than arthritic or neurological involvement, is seen in less than 10% of patients with Lyme disease. Although any layer of the heart may be affected, conduction system involvement is the most common cause of clinical apparent cardiac involvement. Typically, abnormal rhythms are associated with atrioventricular node involvement.

Laboratory Tests and Radiographs

Isolation of *B. burgdorferi* is difficult in most tissues with the exception of the skin, but of obvious importance if positive. It can be accomplished on BDK media.

Evidence of an immunoglobulin M (IgM) humoral response to *B burgdorferi* peaks in about 3 to 4 weeks after infection and is gradually replaced by an IgG response. Nearly all patients will have evidence of a humoral response, detectable by either immunofluorescence or enzyme-linked immunoabsorbent assay. There is considerable variability between laboratories in terms of sensitivity and specificity of results. Moreover, patients with syphilis or other treponemal disorders may manifest false-positive *B burgdorferi* serology. In contrast, patients with only Lyme disease do not have false-positive tests for syphilis. As with many serological tests, Lyme serology should be ordered based upon guidance from the history and physical examination rather than investigating vague or nonspecific symptoms. Questionable serological tests may be confirmed with Western blot analysis.

Other laboratory abnormalities are usually non-specific. There may be a modest elevation of the white blood cell (WBC) count and a minority may have a mild anemia. Erythrocyte sedimentation rates may be normal or slightly elevated. Mild elevation of liver enzymes may be detected in an occasional patient.

Joint fluid is typically inflammatory, with elevation of WBC counts, most of which will be neutrophils. Culture of joint fluid is generally negative, but polymerase chain reaction analysis may provide evidence that the organism is present.

Patients with CNS involvement will usually have a cerebrospinal fluid (CSF) pleocytosis with elevation of synovial fluid protein, but with a normal glucose. CSF cultures are usually not helpful.

Routine joint radiographs are not distinctive and may only demonstrate evidence of soft-tissue swelling or nonspecific erosions in the minority who have an erosive arthritis.

Diagnosis

In endemic areas, a patient who has a classic rash of erythema migrans is virtually diagnostic. Confusion is more often generated when the rash has not appeared or has been forgotten. In a patient presenting with a mono- or oligoarthritis, differential diagnosis should include:

- Reiter's syndrome
- Crystal disease
- Other forms of infectious arthritis.

The course of the disease should discriminate Lyme disease from infectious arthritis. Extra-articular features of Reiter's are not seen with Lyme disease and, of course, crystals are not seen in the synovial fluid in Lyme arthritis.

Similarly, a number of neurological disorders may be brought to mind by the neurological problems associated with Lyme disease. Since the organism is rarely cultured from CSF, meningitis due to Lyme disease must be discriminated from the other forms of aseptic meningitides. History of a tick bite, occurrence in an endemic area, the appearance of erythema migrans, and appropriate serological changes are helpful. In the differential diagnosis of some patients with Lyme disease and neurological symptoms, other disorders may be considered, such as:

- Multiple sclerosis
- Guillain-Barré syndrome
- Bell's palsy.

Management

Prevention is probably the most effective management tool for Lyme disease. Careful and frequent examination of the skin and scalp and removal of any ticks will decrease the likelihood of infection as transmission appears to be linked to the length of time the tick is attached. Tick repellents such as diethyltoluamide are effective. There is no indication for therapy of an asymptomatic patient who has a tick bite or for an asymptomatic seroconverter.

Antibiotic therapy is usually effective in curing Lyme disease. Current recommendations are summarized in Table 8.1. Therapy early in the course is more likely to result in a prompt resolution of symptoms and prevention of sequelae of the disease. Neurological symptoms may occur when oral regimens are administered. Careful attention should be paid to the neurological examination prior to and during the course of therapy, and evidence of abnormalities should prompt consideration for intravenous antibiotic treatment.

Arthritis is treated with:

- Joint rest
- Aspiration of fluid
- Up to 4 weeks of antibiotic therapy.

Based on studies demonstrating the organism in fibroblast and relative resistance to antibiotics, some have suggested a longer course of therapy. No formal studies have been published which address this issue. In those patients who develop resistant arthritis and a proliferative synovitis, an arthroscopic synovectomy has been effective.

Cardiac involvement typically responds rapidly to antibiotics, but 2 to 3 weeks of therapy is the present recommendation. Occasionally, other supportive measures, such as cardiac pacing, may be needed.

Meningitis responds to antibiotic therapy in several days. IV antibiotics are usually recommended for 2 to 3 weeks. In those with long-standing neurological deficits, antibiotic therapy will limit further progression of the disease.

Much has been written about prolonged courses of antibiotics for Lyme disease; there is little data to support such an approach. Most authors have found that the apparent need for prolonged therapy is more likely due to an incorrect diagnosis rather than resistant disease.

Recent vaccination studies suggest that vaccines may be effective in decreasing incidence of Lyme disease.

TABLE 8.1 — CAUSES, DIAGNOSIS AND TREATMENT OF LYME DISEASE

Diagnosis	Suggested Regimens		Comments
	Primary	Alternative	
Tick bite, no symptoms	Antibiotic therapy not indicated	—	—
Early (erythema chronicum migrans)	(Doxycycline 100 mg bid po) or (amoxicillin 500 mg tid po) or (clarithromycin 500 mg bid) × 14-21 d or (cefuroxime axetil 500 mg bid) × 21 d	—	Neurological disease may develop or progress on oral regimens
Carditis	(Ceftriaxone 2 g qd IV) or (cefotaxime 2 g q4h IV) or (Pen G 24 Mu qd IV) × 14-21 d	(Doxycycline 100 mg bid) or (amoxicillin 250-500 mg tid po) × 21 d	Oral regimens only for mild carditis

			Lumbar puncture (LP) suggested to exclude neurological disease. If LP negative, the oral regimen is acceptable; otherwise, the IV regimen should be employed
Facial nerve paralysis (isolated)	(Doxycycline 100 mg bid po) or (amoxicillin 500 mg tid po) × 21-28 d	(Ceftriaxone 2 g qd IV) × 14-28 d	—
Meningitis	(Ceftriaxone 2 g qd IV) × 21 d	(Pen G 20 Mu qd in divided dose IV) or (cefotaxime 2 g q8h IV) × 21 d	—
Arthritis	(Doxycycline 100 mg bid) or (amoxicillin 500 mg qid) po	(Ceftriaxone 2 g qd IV) or (Pen G 20-24 Mu qd IV) × 14-28 d	—
Pregnant women	Choice should not include doxycycline	—	—
Asymptomatic seropositivity	None indicated	—	—

Adapted from: Sanford JP, et al. *The Sanford Guide to Antimicrobial Therapy, 1998.* 1998:41.

8

SUGGESTED READING

Burgdorfer W, Barbour AG, Hayes SF, Benach JL, Granwaldt E, Davis JP. Lyme disease–a tick-borne spirochetosis? *Science*. 1982;216:1317-1319.

Keller D, Koster FT, Marks DH, Hosbach P, Erdile LF, Mays JP. Safety and immunogenicity of a recombinant outer surface protein A Lyme vaccine. *JAMA*. 1994;271:1764-1768.

Logigian EL, Kaplan RF, Steere AC. Chronic neurological manifestations of Lyme disease. *N Engl J Med*. 1990;323:1438-1444.

Sanford JP, Gilbert DN, Moellering RC Jr, Sande MA. *The Sanford Guide to Antimicrobial Therapy, 1998*. 28th ed. Vienna, Va: Antimicrobial Therapy, Inc; 1998:41.

Steere AC, Bartenhagen NH, Craft JE, et al. The early clinical manifestations of Lyme disease. *Ann Intern Med*. 1983;99:76-82.

Steere AC, Malawista SE, Snydman DR. Lyme arthritis: an epidemic of oligoarticular arthritis in children and adults in three Connecticut communities. *Arthritis Rheum*. 1977;20:7-17.

Steere AC, Hutchinson GJ, Rahn DW, et al. Treatment of the early manifestations of Lyme disease. *Ann Intern Med*. 1983;99:22-26.

9 Myositis

As understanding of disorders such as polymyositis has developed, classification schemes have been modified. Myositis and related disorders are now generally referred to under the rubric of inflammatory muscle diseases. As a group, they are still relatively rare and poorly understood disorders. Although there are characteristic differences, they share certain overlapping clinical features and are considered here together.

Pathogenesis

As with many inflammatory disorders of obscure cause, inflammatory muscle diseases are considered as genetically-mediated autoimmune disorders with an otherwise unknown trigger. Human leukocyte antigen (HLA)-DR3, as in many systemic rheumatic disorders, has been demonstrated to be a risk factor for inflammatory muscle disease. Examination of muscle and sera from patients with inflammatory muscle diseases has provided evidence of both cellular and humoral responses that have been proposed as playing a role in the pathogenesis of these disorders. Muscles from patients with polymyositis are infiltrated by CD8+ T cells, most of which are cytotoxic. Analysis of T cell receptors indicate oligoclonality, suggesting at least some specificity of the response. Interestingly, in dermatomyositis, B cells are also often seen, where they are not a prominent component of the infiltrating cells in polymyositis.

Evidence to suggest a humoral role is also indirect. Specific autoantibodies are found in sera of patients with inflammatory muscle disease. Moreover, these antibodies have been shown to penetrate cell membranes and to interact with and inhibit specific enzymatic functions. How and if this relates to the development of myositis is yet to be elucidated.

Occurrence

The disorders considered as inflammatory muscle diseases are relatively rare. Surveys in England in the 1960s suggested a prevalence of 1 in 37,000 and an annual incidence of about 3 per million population. Comparable incidence figures were found in Tennessee over a similar time period for whites, but in black females the incidence was 18 cases per million population per year. Most studies do suggest that the disease is more common in women. Onset is bimodal, with peaks in childhood and middle age.

Clinical Presentation

The most common presentation is the insidious onset of proximal muscle weakness. Patients frequently complain of increasing inability to:
- Rise from a squat or from a chair
- Climb stairs
- Get their hand over their heads to reach objects
- Comb their hair.

Later in the course, distal muscles or pharyngeal muscles may become weak.

In most individuals, specific muscle group testing will establish that there is weakness in predominantly the proximal muscles. The examiner should not be misled by "give-way" weakness, which is more often due to either pain or feigned weakness. In general, muscles are not tender. Patients with dermatomyositis will have characteristic rashes (Figure 9.1), which may temporarily occur in any relationship with the muscle involvement. Gottron's papules (Figure 9.2), a pathognomonic feature of the disease, are erythematous plaques over the extensor surface of the elbows, fingers, and knees, and over the malleoli. The heliotrope rash (Figure 9.3), which is a violaceous discoloration around the eyes, is also a signature finding in dermatomyositis. More nonspecific rashes are also seen, including a photosensitive erythroderma, particularly over the neck, face and upper torso. Subcutaneous calcification can be extensive and varies from an asymptomatic radiographic finding to a pruritic lesion that ulcerates through the skin.

Other organ systems are only occasionally directly involved. Arthralgias and arthritis are not uncommon. When arthritis is present, it generally is nonerosive. Pulmonary interstitial fibrosis is a worrisome finding which may be unresponsive to therapy, and presents with a dry cough and dyspnea on exertion. Of course, individuals with extensive weakness may have problems clearing their secretions and aspiration or atelectasis due to diminished respiratory excursion. An occasional patient may have heart failure or arrythmias due to myocarditis.

Classification of inflammatory muscle diseases have historically been based on associated clinical findings (ie, idiopathic polymyositis, idiopathic dermatomyositis, juvenile myositis, myositis associated with malignancy, and overlap syndromes). As understanding of these disorders has improved, certain histologic and serologic associations have been made (see *Pathogenesis* and *Laboratory Tests and Radiographs* sections, this chapter). The difference between primary polymyositis and dermatomyositis is based on the absence or presence of the characteristic rash described above. Juvenile myositis appears to be much

FIGURE 9.1 — RASH OF DERMATOMYOSITIS

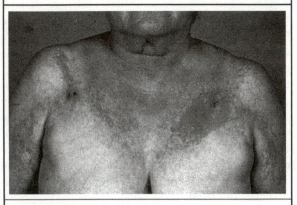

Courtesy of the Arthritis Foundation.

FIGURE 9.2 — GOTTRON'S PAPULES

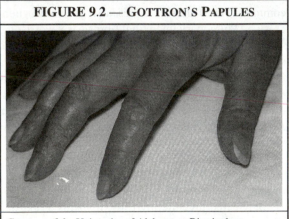

Courtesy of the University of Alabama at Birmingham.

like the adult disease, but children are more likely to have dermatomyositis.

Patients are said to have a myositis overlap syndrome if myositis is part of another inflammatory rheumatic disease. Patients with rheumatoid arthritis, systemic lupus erythematosus, and scleroderma may have myositis as a component of their illnesses.

FIGURE 9.3 — HELIOTROPE RASH OF DERMATOMYOSITIS

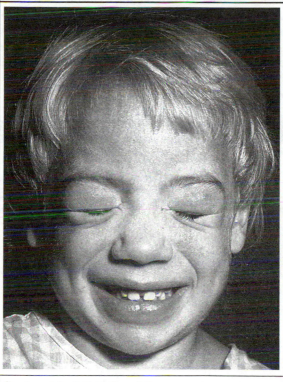

Courtesy of the Arthritis Foundation.

In most patients, the muscle disease is overshadowed by the other features of their disorders.

One clinical impression is that patients with myositis are more likely to develop malignancies. For the most part, these observations were based on anecdotal reports. More recent controlled trials have yielded conflicting results, but there is a suggestion that gastric and ovarian cancers are seen more often in patients with myositis. An often recommended approach is to perform a careful examination and the routine screening tests (eg, mammograms, PAP smears, rectal exam) appropriate for an individual of that particular age. Abnormalities uncovered with these procedures should be vigorously pursued. Outcome of patients with malignancy and myositis is dependent on the outcome of the malignancy. There have been reports of the myositis improving with remission of the cancer, even when there has been surgical extirpation.

Laboratory Tests and Radiographs

Nearly all patients with myositis will have elevation of serum concentrations of muscle cytoplasmic enzymes. Creatine kinase (CK) is the most commonly measured enzyme and is elevated in over 90% of cases. In regenerating muscle, CK-MB band may be released and detectable in the serum when there is no evidence of myocardial disease. Other muscle enzymes, including aldolase, aspartate aminotransferase, alanine aminotransferase, and lactate dehydrogenase, are frequently elevated in patients with active myositis. Other causes of elevated muscle enzymes should always be considered. Trauma, ischemia, and certain drugs may elevate serum levels. Body builders and blacks may have elevated serum levels of muscle enzymes. CK levels are often used to follow therapy, but they should not be used to the exclusion of a history and physical examination.

Other abnormal laboratory tests reflect the systemic inflammation. Erythrocyte sedimentation rate, C-reative protein, white blood cell and platelet counts may be elevated.

Antinuclear antibodies are found in the serum of about 50% or more of patients with myositis. Specific antibodies may be of some utility in defining disease subsets. Jo-1 antibodies (directed against histidyl-tRNA synthetase) and other antisynthetase antibodies are found more often in individuals with active myositis who are also more likely to have interstitial lung disease and perhaps nonerosive arthritis. Antibodies to Mi-2 are seen in some patients with dermatomyositis. Anti-PM-Scl, Ku, and several URNP antibodies seem to select a group of patients with a myositis scleroderma overlap syndrome.

Electromyograms (EMGs) and nerve conduction studies are useful in determining whether there is evidence of a myopathy and in helping to eliminate neuropathic causes of weakness. Typical EMG findings include insertional irritability; short, small, low amplitude polyphasic potentials; and bizarre spikes. Electrical muscle testing is usually performed unilaterally; this aids in identifying specific muscle groups that may be abnormal. Biopsy can be undertaken on the contralateral side, since the EMG itself may induce histological changes which may be confused with myositis.

Muscle biopsies demonstrate degeneration with necrosis, regeneration, and phagocytosis (Figure 9.4).

FIGURE 9.4 — MUSCLE BIOPSY FINDINGS

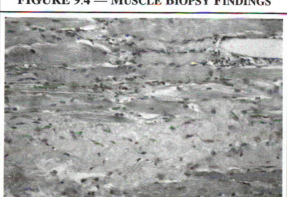

Biopsy from a patient with polymyositis, demonstrating mononuclear cellular infiltration and atrophy.

Courtesy of Arthritis Foundation.

There is frequently perimysial and perivascular infiltration of mononuclear cells. An occasional biopsy may demonstrate a necrotizing vasculitis.

Diagnosis

The diagnosis of an inflammatory myositis is readily made when a patient presents with:
- Proximal muscle weakness
- Elevated levels of muscle enzymes
- Characteristic findings on electrical studies and on muscle biopsy
- The scale of dermatomyositis.

Although developed in 1975, the criteria of Bohan and Peter (Table 9.1) are still of use when considering the diagnosis of inflammatory muscle disease.

However, most patients do not need this extensive evaluation, as a complete history and examination may lead to the discovery of other causes for the patient's weakness. Complaints of weakness are common and are confused with fatigue by many patients. In those with true weakness, it might be discovered through the history that a patient has been exposed to a toxin or used certain drugs that caused elevated muscle enzymes. The fact of a family member with a muscle disease may lead to the diagnosis of a congenital myopathy. Signs and symptoms of hyper- or hypothyroidism may be clues to an endocrine cause of weakness. Careful neurological examination may demonstrate sensory abnormalities which would likely serve to exclude an inflammatory muscle disease. In these situations, other tests will be useful in confirming a specific diagnosis. Examples of other causes of muscle weakness are listed in Table 9.2.

Management

■ Nonpharmacological Therapy

Therapy of patients with inflammatory muscle disease revolves around maneuvers leading to preservation of range of motion and muscle strength and control of inflammation. Rest and range of motion exercises are usually recommended when muscle inflammation is active. As the disease comes under control, progressive strengthening exercises can be employed.

■ Pharmacological Therapy

Corticosteroids remain the mainstay of pharmacological therapy of inflammatory myositis. Therapy is usually initiated with high doses of corticosteroids (1 mg/kg/d or greater of prednisone). Within 1 month of initiating therapy, muscle enzymes usually are dramatically improved. At this time, steroid tapering can begin. Many patients' myositis can eventually be controlled with alternate-day steroids; some individuals will enter apparent remissions, then steroids can be further tapered.

The role of other medications is less clear. Addition of azathioprine or methotrexate may allow for more rapid tapering of the corticosteroids. In open-label studies, cyclosporin A and cyclophosphamide have been used successfully in some patients. Intravenous immunoglobulin has also been used successfully in some patients, but the duration of the response is limited. Recent studies have further demonstrated that either a combination of azathioprine and methotrexate or high dose methotrexate with leucovorin rescue may be useful when other therapies are not effective.

TABLE 9.1 — CRITERIA FOR THE DIAGNOSIS OF POLYMYOSITIS AND DERMATOMYOSITIS*

Criteria	Description
Symmetrical weakness	Weakness of limb-girdle muscles and anterior neck flexors, progressing over weeks to months, with or without dysphagia or respiratory muscle involvement
Muscle biopsy evidence	Evidence of necrosis of type I and II fibers, phagocytosis, regeneration with basophilia, large vesicular sarcolemmal nuclei and prominent nucleoli, atrophy in a perifascicular distribution, variation in fiber size, and an inflammatory exudate, often perivascular
Elevation of muscle enzymes	Elevation in serum of skeletal muscle enzymes, particularly creatine phosphokinase and often aldolase, serum glutamate oxaloacetate, and pyruvate transaminases, and lactate dehydrogenase
Electromyographic evidence	Electromyographic triad of short, small, polyphasic motor units, fibrillations, positive sharp waves, and insertional irritability; and bizarre, high-frequency repetitive discharges

Dermatologic features	A lilac discoloration of the eyelids (heliotrope) with periorbital edema; a scaly, erythematous dermatitis over the dorsum of the hands (especially the metacarpopha-langeal and proximal interphalangeal joints, Gottron's syndrome); and involvement of the knees, elbows, and medial malleoli, as well as the face, neck, and upper torso

* Confidence limits can be defined as follows: For a definite diagnosis of dermatomyositis, three of four criteria plus the rash must be present; for a definite diagnosis of polymyositis, four criteria must be present without the rash. For a probable diagnosis of dermatomyositis, two criteria plus the rash must be present; for a probable diagnosis of poly-myositis, three criteria must be present without the rash. For a possible diagnosis of dermatomyositis, one criterion plus the rash must be present; for a possible diagnosis of polymyositis, two criteria must be present without the rash.

Adapted from: Bohan A, Peter JB. *N Engl J Med.* 1975;292:344-347.

9

TABLE 9.2 — OTHER CAUSES OF MUSCLE WEAKNESS

Metabolic Disorders
- Mitochondrial
- Enzyme deficiencies:
  - Acid maltase
  - Phosphofructokinase
  - Carnitine palmitoyltransferase
- Hyperpyrexia

Drugs/Toxins
- Carbon monoxide
- Clofibrate
- Chloroquine
- Ethanol
- Penicillamine
- Cimetidine
- Lovastatin
- Corticosteroids
- Ipecac
- Zidovudine
- Colchicine

Neurological Disorders
- Amyotrophic lateral sclerosis
- Guillain-Barré syndrome
- Diabetic neuropathies
- Myasthenia gravis

Endocrine
- Thyroid disease (hypo- and hyper-)
- Hypercortisolism
- Hyperparathyroidism
- Hypokalemia

Muscular Dystrophies
- Oculopharyngeal
- Limb-girdle
- Duchenne's syndrome
- Becker's disease
- Fascioscapulohumeral

Cancer Related
- Paraneoplastic
- Hypercalcemia

Infectious
- Viral:
  - Echovirus
  - Coxsackievirus
- Bacterial:
  - Clostridia
  - Staphylococcic
- Protozoal (eg, toxoplasmosis)
- Nematodal (eg, trichinosis)
- May present as myositis or myalgia

9

SUGGESTED READING

Airio A, Pukkala E, Isomäki H. Elevated cancer incidence in patients with dermatomyositis: a population based study. *J Rheumatol.* 1995;22:1300-1303.

Black HR, Quallich H, Gareleck CB. Racial differences in serum creatine kinase levels. *Am J Med.* 1986;81:479-487.

Bohan A, Peter JB. Polymyositis and dermatomyositis (part I and II). *N Engl J Med.* 1975;292:344-347, 403-407.

Bohlmeyer TJ, Wu AH, Perryman MB. Evaluation of laboratory tests as a guide to diagnosis and therapy of myositis. *Rheum Dis Clin North Am.* 1994;20:845-856.

Oddis CV. Therapy of inflammatory myopathy. *Rheum Dis Clin North Am.* 1994;20:899-918.

10   Osteoarthritis

Osteoarthritis (OA) is one of the most common rheumatic disorders. Affecting aging individuals, this disease will manifest signs or symptoms at some time during nearly everyone's life. Based on the recognition that the processes leading to OA are more complicated than simple wearing out of cartilage, terms such as degenerative joint disease have largely been replaced by OA.

Pathogenesis

Cartilage from osteoarthritic joints shows a progression of changes. Damage to the collagen framework leads to expansion of the hydrophilic proteoglycan molecules and increased cartilage water content. Proteoglycan molecules are changed, with a loss of chondroitin sulfate relative to keratin sulfate. Perhaps in an attempt to repair the damaged cartilage, the number of chondrocytes increases, as does their metabolic activity. However, there is a corresponding increase in production of degradative enzymes. Although there may be a component of wear in mediating cartilage degradation, most data suggest that the cathepsins and metalloproteases, such as collagenase, gelatinase, and stromelysin, are responsible for cartilage resorption. More recently, it has been noted that synovial tissue is increased in some patients with OA, and there is expression of cytokines such as interleukin (IL)-1, which increases expression of degradative proteases and likely enhances chondrocyte degradative activity.

Despite the attempts by chondrocytes to increase cartilage synthesis, the balance is shifted and there is progressive loss of cartilage macromolecules. Eventually this becomes apparent, initially as microscopic fissuring and later as grossly visible changes, including cartilage ulceration. The collagen matrix is eventually lost, marking irreversible damage. Accompanying these changes are increases in subjacent bone. Often, this bony increase occurs at the joint margin, leading to the development of osteophytes or spurs.

Based on observations of processes where OA develops secondarily, a number of factors have been recognized as having a role in its development:

- Trauma, particularly when there is disruption of cartilage, rapidly leads to the development of osteoarthritis.
- Anterior cruciate resection, followed by weight bearing, also rapidly leads to OA of the knee.
- Repetitive compressive stress to cartilage leads to degradation (more normal loading, such as with long-distance running, does not seem to increase the risk of OA).
- Disorders associated with joint inflammation and injury, (eg, rheumatoid arthritis [RA] or septic arthritis) alteration in the compressibility of cartilage (eg, acromegaly, ochronosis), or disorders that alter joint sensation (eg, syringomyelia or diabetes mellitus).

A number of these factors have been postulated as causes of primary OA, such as:

- Subtle mechanical abnormalities, which are thought to be responsible for most cases of primary OA of the hip.
- A point mutation in the type II collagen gene, which has been shown to be related to severe familial OA, leading to speculation of subtle changes in this or other joint macromolecules.

- Stiffness of the subchondral bone and decreased effectiveness of the energy-absorbing musculature around the joint.

Occurrence

By the age of 55, over 80% of the population will have radiographic evidence of OA. Fortunately, many will not be symptomatic, but a number of prevalence estimates have suggested that as many as one half of those middle aged or older will have some symptoms; the older the population, the higher the prevalence. OA of the knee occurs in women more often than in men, whereas OA of the hip is as frequent in men as in women. Black women seem to have OA of the knee more often than white women, but this observation may be confounded by other risk factors.

A number of other distinct risk factors have been linked to the development of OA. Based on the Framingham study, obesity is a clear risk factor for development of OA of the knee, particularly in women. Moreover, the risk increases when those with severe OA are evaluated. Those family members with OA of the hands are at increased risk of developing OA elsewhere. Genetic factors that constitute this risk, if any, have yet to be determined. Major joint trauma has been linked to the development of OA. Similarly, vocations seem to be linked to OA, including jackhammer operators, boxers, and shipyard workers. In contrast, those who have been able to run long distances for long periods of time do not seem to be at an increased risk for developing OA.

Clinical Features

The major manifestation of OA is pain. Since articular cartilage is not innervated, pain due to OA is thought to emanate from:

119

- Subchondral bone
- Impinged nerves
- A stretched capsule or other local structures.

Typically, pain occurs initially with joint use and resolves with rest. The pain is perceived as deep and aching, although there may be associated bony tenderness.

Patients often note periods of remissions or exacerbations which may last months. With progression, symptoms may become more severe and continuous, and pain develops even during rest or sleep. In others, there may be periods of resolution or stability of joint symptoms. OA of the hand is notorious for sequentially involving many of the proximal interphalangeal (PIP) or distal interphalangeal (DIP) joints, but eventually becoming pain free. Stiffness or gelling may develop after joint rest and usually resolves rapidly, generally within about 15 to 30 minutes. Cracking or popping of the joint is often noted with motion. In the knee, a sense of instability or giving way may be noted, particularly on uneven ground. Joints may lock transiently and then painfully give way. As bony changes develop in the joint, range of motion may become limited.

Joint examination may demonstrate:
- Crepitus with motion
- Bony tenderness
- Enlargement.

The enlargement of the DIP and PIP joints is called Heberden's and Bouchard's nodes, respectively (Figure 10.1). With cartilage loss, joint instability may develop, and is particularly common in the knee.

Primary OA involves mainly the:
- DIP, PIP, and first carpometacarpal joints of the hand (Figure 10.2)
- Lower lumbar and cervical spine

FIGURE 10.1 — HEBERDEN'S AND BOUCHARD'S NODES

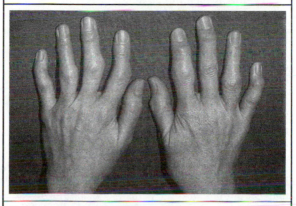

Courtesy of Syntex Laboratories, Inc.

FIGURE 10.2 — OSTEOARTHRITIS OF THE DISTAL AND PROXIMAL INTERPHALANGEAL JOINTS

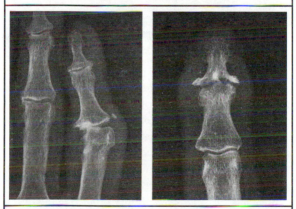

Left: Radiograph illustrating joint space loss, subchondral sclerosis, and osteophytes. *Right*: Typical chevroning seen in the distal interphalangeal joints.

Courtesy of Gower Medical Publishing Ltd.

- Hips
- Knees
- First metatarsophalangeal.

Apparent OA of the glenohumeral joint, elbow, wrist, or talonavicular joint should prompt a search for secondary causes, as these are atypical joints for primary OA.

Pain from involved joints is usually felt diffusely within the joint, however, pain from some joints is often radiated. OA of the hip is usually felt as buttock, groin, or even knee pain, and should not be confused with knee disease. Internal rotation of the hip may reproduce symptoms. Lumbar spine involvement is noted as buttock or thigh pain. Cervical spine involvement may be noted in the neck, shoulder or down the arm. With both cervical and lumbar spine OA, impingement of a nerve root leads to pain along the distribution of the nerve. Knee OA is usually felt in the knee, but may be noted initially when going down hills or stairs.

Laboratory Tests and Radiographs

Routine blood tests are typically normal in patients with OA. Occasionally, laboratory tests are useful if a secondary cause of OA is being considered, or as a monitor for drug toxicity during therapy. Synovial fluid is usually straw colored with only a modest increase in white blood cells, generally no more than 1000 to 2000 cells/mm^3. Other abnormalities, such as crystals or higher synovial fluid blood cell counts, suggest that a secondary process is operative.

Radiographs are often useful in assisting with the diagnosis and occasionally with management. However, the correlation between symptoms and radiographic changes is poor. Early, there is loss of joint space, which is best determined when radiographs are obtained while the patient is bearing weight (Figure 10.3). Later, subchondral sclerosis and bony eburnation will be visible. Other imaging modalities, such as magnetic resonance imaging, may provide better cartilage visualization and may be useful in clinical trials.

Diagnosis

The diagnosis is readily made when there is:
- Weight-bearing pain in a typical joint
- Characteristic examination
- Radiographic findings.

The American College of Rheumatology (ACR) has established diagnostic criteria (Table 10.1).

Rheumatoid factor and antinuclear antibodies (ANA) occur commonly in the general normal population. Occasionally, physicians may be misled by overreliance on these laboratory tests. A patient with OA involving the PIP and DIP joints who coincidentally has a positive rheumatoid factor should not be mistakenly thought to have RA; or a person with OA and a positive ANA should not mistakenly be thought to have lupus. More importantly, secondary causes of OA should not be overlooked, particularly when the joints involved or the course of the disease are atypical.

Management

The goals of therapy of OA are to:
- Maintain joint mobility and function
- Limit pain.

Although, there is no evidence that presently available therapies will reverse the histological changes of OA, much can be done toward accomplishing the

FIGURE 10.3 — OSTEOARTHRITIS OF THE HIP AND KNEE JOINTS

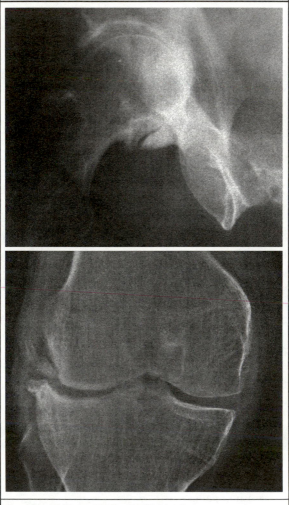

Courtesy of Gower Medical Publishing Ltd.

therapeutic goals. Unfortunately, overreliance on pharmacological measures with the exclusion on other modalities often results in a less than optimum outcome.

Discussions of therapy with patients with OA generally focus on three areas, each not exclusive of the others, including:
- Limiting joint loading
- Improving muscle strength and maintaining range of motion
- Pain relief.

■ **Nonpharmacological Therapy**
Limiting Joint Loading

Limiting joint loading may simply involve minor activity modifications. Some examples include:
- Those with OA of the lumbar spine may be instructed on proper lifting techniques.
- Those with OA of the knee may be instructed to avoid stairs and squatting down.
- OA of the hand may be improved with a number of utensils or assistive devices which limit stress of those joints.
- When there is lower extremity involvement or OA of the lumbosacral spine, weight loss is important.
- Cervical spine disease may be improved with a soft cervical collar worn at night.

Patient involvement in these discussions will often pinpoint particularly bothersome activities.

Muscle Strengthening

Muscle strengthening exercises are useful in:
- Improving joint stability
- Decreasing muscle spasm
- Increasing aerobic capacity.

TABLE 10.1 — CRITERIA FOR THE CLASSIFICATION OF OSTEOARTHRITIS OF THE HAND, HIP AND KNEE

*Classification Criteria for Osteoarthritis of the Hand**

Hand pain, aching, or stiffness and three or four of the following features:
- Hard tissue enlargement of two or more of 10 selected joints
- Hard tissue enlargement of two or more DIP joints
- Fewer than three swollen MCP joints
- Deformity of at least one of 10 selected joints

Classification Criteria for Osteoarthritis of the Hip[†]

Hip pain and at least two of the following three features:
- ESR < 20 mm/h
- Radiographic femoral or acetabular osteophytes
- Radiographic joint-space narrowing (superior, axial, and/or medial)

Classification Criteria for Idiopathic Osteoarthritis of the Knee

Clinical and Laboratory[‡]
Knee pain plus at least five of the following nine features:
- Age > 50 years
- Stiffness < 30 min
- Crepitus
- Bony tenderness
- Bony enlargement
- No palpable warmth
- ESR < 40 mm/h
- RF < 1:40
- SF OA

Clinical and Radiographic[§]
Knee pain plus at least one of the following three features:
- Age < 50 years
- Stiffness < 30 min
- Crepitus + osteophytes

Clinical[¶]

Knee pain plus at least three of the following six features:
- Age > 50 years
- Stiffness < 30 min
- Crepitus
- Bony tenderness
- Bony enlargement
- No palpable warmth

Abbreviations: DIP, distal interphalangeal; MCP, metacarpophalangeal; ESR, erythrocyte sedimentation rate (Westergren method); RF, rheumatoid factor; SF OA, synovial fluid signs of osteoarthritis.

* The 10 selected joints are the second and third DIP, the second and third proximal interphalangeal, and the first carpometacarpal joints of both hands. This classification method yields a sensitivity of 94% and a specificity of 87%.

† This classification method yields a sensitivity of 89% and a specificity of 91%.

‡ This classification method yields a sensitivity of 92% and a specificity of 75%.

§ This classification method yields a sensitivity of 91% and a specificity of 86%.

¶ This classification method yields a sensitivity of 95% and a specificity of 69%. Alternative for the clinical category would be four of six, which is 84% sensitive and 89% specific.

Reprinted from: Altman R, et al. *Arthritis Rheum.* 1986;29:1039-1049. Altman R, et al. *Arthritis Rheum.* 1990;33:1601-1610. Altman R, et al. *Arthritis Rheum.* 1991;34:505-514.

Even in patients with lower-extremity OA, walking may be useful, particularly if prescribed in a graded fashion. Patients quickly learn how far they can walk without increasing pain. Further activity past this point is counterproductive. Those unable to walk may tolerate a stationary bicycle or participate in water aerobic programs.

Strengthening of the quadriceps may diminish pain due to OA of the knee. For example, while patients are sitting, one leg can be held in extension by contracting the quadriceps. This is continued until the quadricep muscle is fatigued, at which time the other leg is extended. Leg lifts and other exercises that strengthen abdominal muscles may improve low-back pain. Simple range of motion exercises, with rotation, lateral bending, and flexion and extension, may improve OA of the cervical spine.

The therapies discussed above may well limit pain and no other therapy may be needed. However, frequently this is not the case, and other therapies are necessary. Prior to changes in therapy, it is worthwhile to make certain that the pain is due to OA. Frequently, periarticular sources of pain are cited as reasons for therapeutic failures. In contrast, appropriate recognition that knee pain is not due to OA but rather to anserine bursitis, or hip pain is due to trochanteric bursitis, may make treatment simpler and more effective.

Topical Therapies

Simple application of either heat or cold may be soothing to some patients. There is little science toward the recommendation of either of these, and generally the choice is based upon empiric results. Capsaicin cream is effective in diminishing pain due to OA. This compound depletes peripheral nerve substance P by releasing it and blocking its reuptake. It generates a sensation of warmth at the site of application, which some patients find soothing, but others irritating. The sensation returns with heating the area or after exertion. Inadvertent application to mucosal membranes is particularly irritating.

■ **Pharmacological Therapy**

Oral agents used for treatment of OA include:
- Acetaminophen

- Nonsteroidal anti-inflammatory drugs (NSAIDs)
- Centrally-acting analgesics (eg, tramadol)
- Opioid analgesics (eg, propoxyphene, codeine, oxycodone).

There is no role for systemic corticosteroids in the treatment of OA.

Acetaminophen

The ACR guidelines for the treatment of hip and knee OA recommend that acetaminophen in a daily dose of up to 4000 mg be used as the first oral agent for treating the symptomatic patient with OA (see Figures 10.4 and 10.5). In short-term studies of patients with chronic knee pain and moderately severe radiograph changes of OA, it has been demonstrated that acetaminophen is as effective as ibuprofen in decreasing pain. The presence of clinical signs of synovitis was not predictive of a better response to treatment with an anti-inflammatory dose of ibuprofen than with acetaminophen. Other studies have further indicated that analgesics (ie, acetaminophen-propoxyphene) are as effective in controlling pain as NSAIDs.

At doses up to 4000 mg/d, good analgesic responses are noted. Side effects are rare and generally mild. Massive overdoses of acetaminophen may cause hepatic toxicity, however, this has generally been seen with daily doses exceeding 10 g, or 2 and one half times the maximum recommended therapeutic dose for adults. An interaction with alcohol and liver disease is a concern but appears to be linked primarily to chronic alcohol abusers who use acetaminophen in excess of recommended levels. Nonetheless, patients who regularly consume alcohol should be discouraged from regular use of any analgesic.

10

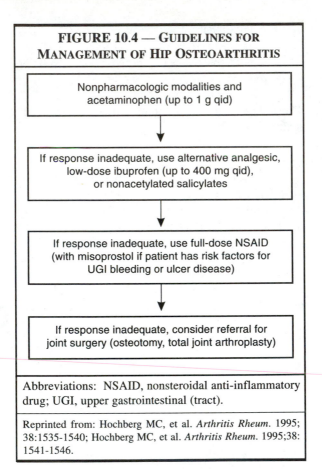

FIGURE 10.4 — GUIDELINES FOR MANAGEMENT OF HIP OSTEOARTHRITIS

Nonpharmacologic modalities and acetaminophen (up to 1 g qid)

↓

If response inadequate, use alternative analgesic, low-dose ibuprofen (up to 400 mg qid), or nonacetylated salicylates

↓

If response inadequate, use full-dose NSAID (with misoprostol if patient has risk factors for UGI bleeding or ulcer disease)

↓

If response inadequate, consider referral for joint surgery (osteotomy, total joint arthroplasty)

Abbreviations: NSAID, nonsteroidal anti-inflammatory drug; UGI, upper gastrointestinal (tract).

Reprinted from: Hochberg MC, et al. *Arthritis Rheum.* 1995; 38:1535-1540; Hochberg MC, et al. *Arthritis Rheum.* 1995;38: 1541-1546.

■ Nonsteroidal Anti-inflammatory Drugs

Historically, NSAIDs were the initial agents chosen by physicians for the treatment of OA. However, several studies indicate that they are no more effective than acetaminophen in relieving pain. These compounds inhibit cyclooxygenase (COX)-1 and 2. This has been based on the perception that the anti-inflammatory effects of NSAIDs may provide additional benefit. As noted above, in terms of pain relief, there is little supporting data. There have been *ex vivo* re-

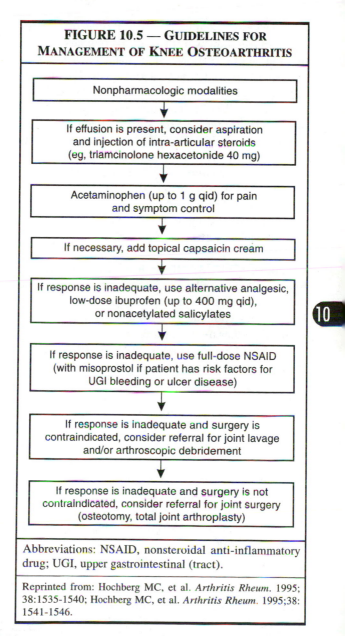

FIGURE 10.5 — GUIDELINES FOR MANAGEMENT OF KNEE OSTEOARTHRITIS

Nonpharmacologic modalities

↓

If effusion is present, consider aspiration and injection of intra-articular steroids (eg, triamcinolone hexacetonide 40 mg)

↓

Acetaminophen (up to 1 g qid) for pain and symptom control

↓

If necessary, add topical capsaicin cream

↓

If response is inadequate, use alternative analgesic, low-dose ibuprofen (up to 400 mg qid), or nonacetylated salicylates

↓

If response is inadequate, use full-dose NSAID (with misoprostol if patient has risk factors for UGI bleeding or ulcer disease)

↓

If response is inadequate and surgery is contraindicated, consider referral for joint lavage and/or arthroscopic debridement

↓

If response is inadequate and surgery is not contraindicated, consider referral for joint surgery (osteotomy, total joint arthroplasty)

Abbreviations: NSAID, nonsteroidal anti-inflammatory drug; UGI, upper gastrointestinal (tract).

Reprinted from: Hochberg MC, et al. *Arthritis Rheum*. 1995; 38:1535-1540; Hochberg MC, et al. *Arthritis Rheum*. 1995;38: 1541-1546.

10

ports suggesting that certain NSAIDs decrease cartilage turnover, however, there is no credible evidence that similar observations can be made *in vivo*. Short-term studies have demonstrated that NSAIDs are better than placebo for controlling the pain of OA. However, most studies indicate that long-term control by the use of a single NSAID occurs infrequently. The combination of NSAIDs and acetaminophen appears to be more effective than NSAIDs alone.

When a decision is made to treat OA with an NSAID, the side effects of these medications must be considered, including:

- Gastrointestinal (GI) side effects
- Renal side effects.

Gastrointestinal side effects occur in about 20% of treated patients and include perforation, ulcers and bleeding in about 1% to 2% of patients. Patients more likely to develop side effects include the elderly and those with other medical problems.

Among elderly patients, the rate of hospitalization for peptic ulcer disease is 4 times greater among NSAID users than for those not taking an NSAID. The risk of hospitalization increases with the dose, rising from 4 cases per 1000 population for those not taking an NSAID to more than 40 per 1000 for those using the largest NSAID doses. The disease of patients thought to require NSAIDs and who develop GI side effects sometimes can be effectively managed by the addition of misoprostol or proton-pump inhibitors. These additional agents may be considered in those patients who are at high risk for developing signficiant GI complications.

Renal side effects are more likely to develop in patients who have underlying renal or cardiac disease or who are undergoing other hemodynamic compromise. Given the present state of knowledge, a prudent course would be to prescribe the smallest

132

effective dose. Further, when the disease becomes quiescent, it is reasonable to either decrease the dose or discontinue the medication until symptoms reappear.

Presently available NSAIDs inhibit the activity of both of the known isoforms of the COX enzymes. COX-1 is present in platelets and gastric mucosa, whereas both are found in synovium of patients with OA. It has been thought that inhibition of COX-1 is associated with the most important side effects of NSAIDs. Selective inhibition of COX-2 should result in efficacy but decreased side effects.

■ COX-2 Targeted NSAIDs

The first available COX-2 targeted agent, celecoxib, has been shown to be as effective as naproxen and other NSAIDs in the treatment of OA. In a 12-week multicenter, placebo-controlled, double-blind study of 1003 patients with symptomatic osteoarthritis of the knee, treatment with celecoxib resulted in significant improvement in the signs and symptoms of osteoarthritis (Figure 10.6). Significant pain relief occurred within the first 2 days of treatment, with maximal anti-inflammatory and analgesic effect evident within 2 weeks. Benefit was sustained throughout the 12-week trial.

Several studies have further demonstrated that GI tolerability of celecoxib is comparable to placebo and significantly better than naproxen. Since its introduction, there has been extensive experience with this medication and post-marketing surveys representing over 340,000 patient years of use remarkably suggest that the rate of significant GI complications with celecoxib (ie, ulcers, perforation, and bleeding) are very low and comparable to background rates. Interestingly, celecoxib, perhaps because of its GI tolerability, has been shown to improve quality of life mea-

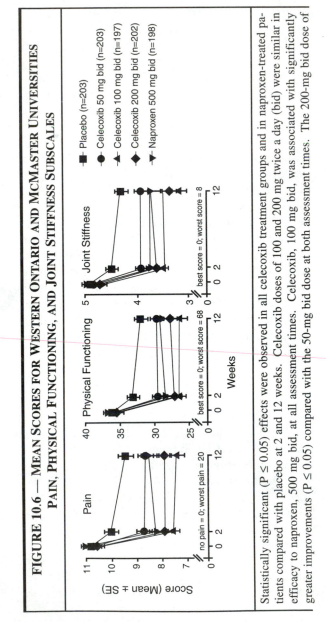

FIGURE 10.6 — MEAN SCORES FOR WESTERN ONTARIO AND MCMASTER UNIVERSITIES PAIN, PHYSICAL FUNCTIONING, AND JOINT STIFFNESS SUBSCALES

Statistically significant (P ≤ 0.05) effects were observed in all celecoxib treatment groups and in naproxen-treated patients compared with placebo at 2 and 12 weeks. Celecoxib doses of 100 and 200 mg twice a day (bid) were similar in efficacy to naproxen, 500 mg bid, at all assessment times. Celecoxib, 100 mg bid, was associated with significantly greater improvements (P ≤ 0.05) compared with the 50-mg bid dose at both assessment times. The 200-mg bid dose of celecoxib was statistically superior ($P \leq 0.05$) to the 50-mg bid dose in Western Ontario and McMaster Universities (WOMAC) pain subscale at both assessment times and at the 2-week assessment in the WOMAC physical function subscale. A significant ($P \leq 0.05$) difference between naproxen-treated patients and patients in the celecoxib 50-mg bid treatment group was detected only in the WOMAC pain subscale at the week 2 assessment.

Bensen WG, et al. *Mayo Clin Proc.* 1999;74:1100.

sures more than naproxen in older patients with osteoarthritis.

Further, celecoxib does not interfere with platelet function or increase bleeding time. Coupled with the data demonstrating GI tolerability makes this compound a consideration in the patient on warfarin who has uncontrolled OA.

Rofecoxib is a newer agent which also preferentially inhibits the COX-2 enzyme. It has been shown to be as effective as conventional NSAIDs and it, too, has a better GI safety profile than non-selective cyclooxygenase inhibitors. Based on a meta-analysis of several OA studies, perforations, ulcers, and GI bleeding occurred less frequently with rofecoxib than older NSAIDs (Figure 10.7). Rofecoxib, like celecoxib, does not interfere with platelet function. Overall, patients treated with these COX-2 selective agents might be expected to require fewer GI medications and procedures.

■ Other Pharmacological Therapies

Oral narcotics are occasionally prescribed for individuals whose pain is not controlled by other means. In addition to agents such as codeine and propoxyphene, tramadol is available for treatment of pain. Tramadol is not classified as a narcotic, but does bind the opioid receptors. Abuse potential is low. Due to tramadol's inhibition of norepinephrine and serotonin, patients who are receiving selective serotonin reuptake inhibitors, tricyclic antidepressants, or monoamine oxidase inhibitors should not receive tramadol. The drug has been approved for management of moderately severe pain and has been shown to be effective in patients with osteoarthritis. A 100-mg dose of tramadol provides pain relief superior to 60 mg of codeine, but is comparable to the combination of 650 mg of acetaminophen with 100 mg of propoxyphene.

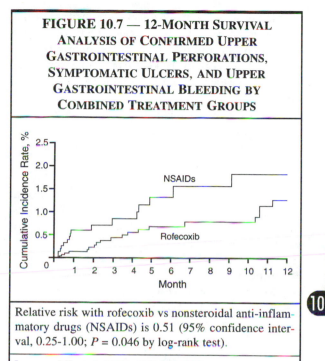

FIGURE 10.7 — 12-MONTH SURVIVAL ANALYSIS OF CONFIRMED UPPER GASTROINTESTINAL PERFORATIONS, SYMPTOMATIC ULCERS, AND UPPER GASTROINTESTINAL BLEEDING BY COMBINED TREATMENT GROUPS

Relative risk with rofecoxib vs nonsteroidal anti-inflammatory drugs (NSAIDs) is 0.51 (95% confidence interval, 0.25-1.00; $P = 0.046$ by log-rank test).

Langman MJ, et al. *JAMA*. 1999;282:1932.

With all these medications, habituation is a potential problem.

Finally, intra-articular therapy may be of benefit in some patients. Intra-articular corticosteroids provide rapid and prolonged pain relief. In many patients, particularly those with OA of the knee, pain returns within 1 or 2 weeks. The systemic side effects of repeated injections at this interval are unacceptable. However, patients' disease may be managed long term if injections are only needed less frequently than every 3 months.

Joint lavage is another therapy for OA which is undergoing a reanalysis. Reports of improvement after arthroscopy for OA of the knee are likely due to simple lavage. The mechanisms responsible for this improvement have not been determined; it has been speculated that removal of cartilage debris may be beneficial. Lavage of the knee can be undertaken using local anesthetics and large-bore needles or with office arthroscopic equipment.

A final intra-articular therapy for OA involves the administration of large molecular weight agents such as hyaluronic acid. Recommended courses involve several injections administered over the course of 1 to 2 weeks, followed by periodic injections. Most reports indicate that pain is decreased after several weeks and may last for several months. The magnitude of the improvement is comparable to that produced by intra-articular corticosteroids.

■ Summary

Many patients who are compliant with the nonpharmacological interventions can be managed with either topical agents or acetaminophen. Those who continue to have unacceptable pain, and other nonarticular features have been excluded, may benefit from the addition of low-dose NSAIDs. Should this not be effective, agents such as tramadol or low doses of codeine may be useful. Finally, incrementing the dose of NSAIDs may result in pain relief. As with other rheumatic diseases, pain due to OA may exacerbate and remit. Additional medications required during an exacerbation may be tapered during the more quiescent phases. Patients failing all these interventions may be candidates for surgical intervention.

Surgical Therapy

A number of surgical procedures may be useful in the treatment of OA. In carefully selected patients,

procedures such as a tibial osteotomy may be helpful. In contrast, total joint replacement of the hip or
knee is one of the leading advancements in the therapy
of OA. Even with advanced changes on radiographs,
a patient may have limited symptoms. Joint arthroplasty is usually reserved for the patient whose pain
due to OA is not otherwise controlled. In that setting, the vast majority will benefit from pain relief.
Present expectation is that a joint arthroplasty performed today should last at least 15 years.

SUGGESTED READING

Altman R, Alarcon G, Appelrouth D, et al. The American College
of Rheumatology criteria for the classification and reporting of osteoarthritis of the hand. *Arthritis Rheum*. 1990;33:1601-1610.

Altman R, Alarcon G, Appelrouth D, et al. The American College
of Rheumatology criteria for the classification and reporting of osteoarthritis of the hip. *Arthritis Rheum*. 1991;34:505-514.

Altman R, Asch E, Block D, et al. Development of criteria for the
classification and reporting of osteoarthritis. Classification of osteoarthritis of the knee. *Arthritis Rheum*. 1986;29:1039-1049.

Barkin RL. Focus on tramadol: centrally acting analgesic for moderate to moderately severe pain. *Hospital Formulary*. 1995;30:321-
325.

Bensen WG, Agrawal N, Zhao S, et al. Upper gastrointestinal tolerability of celecoxib: a Cox-2 specific inhibitor, compared to
naproxen and placebo. *Arthritis Rheum*. 1999;42:S142.

Bensen WG, Fiechtner JJ, McMillen JI, et al. Treatment of osteoarthritis with celecoxib, a cyclooxygenase-2 inhibitor: a randomized
controlled trial. *Mayo Clin Proc*. 1999;74:1095-1105.

Bradley JD, Brandt KD, Katz BP, Kalasinski LA, Ryan SI. Comparison of an anti-inflammatory dose of ibuprofen, an analgesic
dose of ibuprofen, and acetaminophen in the treatment of patients
with osteoarthritis of the knee. *N Engl J Med*. 1991;325:87-91.

10

Bradley JD, Brandt KD, Katz BP, Kalasinski LA, Ryan SI. Treatment of knee osteoarthritis: relationship of clinical features of joint inflammation to the response to a nonsteroidal anti-inflammatory drug or pure analgesic. *J Rheumatol*. 1992;19:1950-1954.

Griffin MR, Piper JM, Daughtery JR, Snowden M, Ray WA. Nonsteroidal anti-inflammatory drug use and increased risk for peptic ulcer disease in elderly persons. *Ann Intern Med*. 1991;114:257-263.

Hochberg MC, Altman RD, Brandt KD, et al. Guidelines for the medical management of osteoarthritis. Part I. Osteoarthritis of the hip. American College of Rheumatology. *Arthritis Rheum*. 1995;38:1535-1540.

Hochberg MC, Altman RD, Brandt KD, et al. Guidelines for the medical management of osteoarthritis. Part II. Osteoarthritis of the knee. American College of Rheumatology. *Arthritis Rheum*. 1995;38:1541-1546.

Langman MJ, Jensen DM, Watson DJ, et al. Adverse upper gastrointestinal effects of rofecoxib compared with NSAIDs. *JAMA*. 1999;282:1929-1933.

Singh G, Ramey D, Triadafilopoulos G. Early experience with selective Cox-2 inhibitors, safety profile in over 340,000 patient years of use. *Arthritis Rheum*. 1999;42:S296.

Stamp J, Rhind V, Haslock I. A comparison of nefopam and flurbiprofen in the treatment of osteoarthritis. *Br J Clin Pract*. 1989;43:24-26.

Sunshine A. New clinical experience with tramadol. *Drugs*. 1994;47(suppl 1):S1-8–S1-18.

Watson D, Harper S, Zhar P, Bolognese J, Simon T, Seidenberg B.Treatment with rofecoxib required less gastrointestinal co-medication and fewer GI procedures than nonspecific cyclooxygenase inhibitiors. *Arthritis Rheum*. 1999;42:S403.

Zhao S, Dedhiya S, Verburg K, Fort J, Osterhaus J. Celecoxib improves health related quality of life of elderly patients with osteoarthritis. *Arthritis Rheum*. 1999;42:S296.

11

Polymyalgia Rheumatica and Giant Cell Arteritis

Polymyalgia rheumatica (PMR) and giant cell arteritis (GCA) are two related inflammatory disorders which often coexist and share some clinical features. In many situations, the symptoms of PMR may be present at the time the diagnosis of GCA is made. Remarkable for their ethnic clustering, these are also disorders of older adults. Although their etiology is unknown, they may represent a continuum of the same disorder.

Pathogenesis

The causes of either PMR or GCA are not known, but there are a number of clues. The ethnic clustering (see below) suggests that these disorders have a genetic association. Approximately one half of patients with GCA express human leukocyte antigen (HLA)-DR4. Even more interestingly, a shared sequence mapped to the antigen-binding site of HLA-DR molecules suggest that there may be specific antigen-binding sequences linked to GCA. Similar genetic associations have been noted in PMR.

Based on the pathology of the lesions in GCA (which includes macrophages; some of which form the characteristic giant cells) and CD4+ T cells, it has been hypothesized that the inciting event (yet to be discovered) is inefficiently resolved. Furthermore, there is evidence indicating that macrophages and T cells in the lesional vessels are activated and producing inflammatory cytokines consistent with a delayed hypersensitivity response. Of note, similar macrophage cytokines and the T cell cytokine interleukin (IL)-2 are found in temporal artery specimens that appear normal under a microscope and that come from patients with PMR.

Despite these intriguing observations, the specific antigens and reasons for the disease localization has not been determined.

Occurrence

The prevalence of PMR and GCA depends upon the geographic location where they occur, and reflects the ethnic background of the local population. The prevalence is highest in those individuals with Scandinavian descent. PMR and GCA are unusual in blacks and Orientals. Women develop this disorder about 3 times as often as men. Older individuals are almost exclusively affected, and PMR or GCA are almost never considerations in individuals under 50 years of age.

Epidemiological studies from northern Europe discovered that the incidence of GCA was over 20 cases per 100,000 annually. Comparable incidence rates were noted in a study in Minnesota, an area of the United States where a Scandinavian heritage is common and where it was also noted that the prevalence in those over 50 years of age was over 200 cases per 100,000 population. In contrast, studies performed in Tennessee in the 1970s and in Texas in the 1980s reported that the annual incidence was under 2 per 100,000, likely reflecting differences in the ethnic composition of the states.

Studies evaluating the occurrence of PMR are more difficult due to the less distinctive clinical presentation. In endemic areas, incidence rates range from 20 to over 50 per 100,000 in those over 50 years of age. Other studies in southern Europe reported an incidence of about 13 per 100,000. Interestingly though, based on a telephone survey in England, it has been reported that over 3% of the population over 65 years of age has symptoms suggestive of PMR, suggesting that this disease may be significantly underdiagnosed.

Clinical Presentation

Symptoms of pain and stiffness in the proximal muscles of the shoulders, neck, and hips in an elderly individual should alert the clinician to consider PMR. Symptoms are usually relatively acute in onset, typically symmetrical, and often associated with prolonged morning stiffness. Other systemic symptoms, including low-grade fever and malaise, are sometimes seen. Synovitis of large joints has been demonstrated in some patients, but involvement of small joints is unusual.

About 50% of patients found to have GCA will have a history suggestive of PMR. About 80% of patients with GCA will have headache. Often, the headache is lancinating, but may be dull or throbbing. Often, the pain is unilateral and scalp or temporal artery tenderness may be noted. On questioning, some patients report jaw fatigue when chewing.

The most feared complications of GCA are related to ischemia in the distribution of the involved vessels. Visual impairment due to involvement of the posterior ciliary arteries is the most common, but retinal artery involvement does occur. Associated symptoms include scotoma, amaurosis fugax, and blindness. Involvement of other vessels, particularly those emanating from the aortic arch, leads to symptoms of transient ischemic attacks, strokes or upper extremity claudication.

Laboratory Tests and Radiographs

Both PMR and GCA are associated by a striking elevation of acute phase proteins. Erythrocyte sedimentation rates (ESRs) are elevated, often to greater than 100 mm/h, and C-reactive protein is elevated. IL-6, one of the most potent stimulators of hepatic acute phase protein synthesis, is also elevated (although its measurement has not been demonstrated to be useful in a clinical setting). Other laboratory findings are reflective of the acute phase response; there is anemia of chronic diseases and elevated platelet counts.

Patients with GCA have characteristic changes on biopsy, usually of the temporal artery. Mononuclear cells often infiltrate all layers of the vessel. Multinucleated giant cells may be present and are often contiguous with the elastic lamina. The elastic lamina is generally disrupted. These lesions are often discontinuous and, if too small a section is analyzed or too few sections made, a false-negative result may ensue.

Diagnosis

The diagnosis of PMR is generally considered when an older patient presents with soreness and stiffness of the shoulder and pelvic girdle. This, coupled with the finding of an ESR, almost always > 50 mm/h, is suggestive of the disease unless other causes are found. In some patients, a therapeutic trial of prednisone may be helpful. Even daily doses as low as 20 mg or less of prednisone results in dramatic and prompt improvement, which may be seen as early as the day after steroids are started. Steroid responsiveness is so reproducible that, if there is not such a response, the diagnosis should be reconsidered.

Occasionally, other inflammatory disorders, such as rheumatoid arthritis (RA) or a seronegative spondyloarthropathy (SNSA), may be confused with PMR. Patients with RA will have peripheral joint synovitis in addition to stiffness. Patients with an SNSA may have axial involvement, or more characteristically, extra-articular features.

Development of new headaches in an older patient who has an unexplained, markedly elevated ESR prompts consideration of GCA. The American College of Rheumatology has developed diagnostic criteria (Table 11.1). Although the diagnosis can certainly be made without histological confirmation, a confirmatory biopsy reduces subsequent confusion if therapeutic responses are not consistent with expectations, particularly when the consideration is whether to continue cortiocosteroids. When the biopsy is performed, an extended piece should be obtained and multiple sections evaluated. If the clinical suspicion is high and the initial biopsy is negative, a contralateral biopsy will demonstrate diagnostic changes in about 10% of further cases.

A more controversial consideration is whether to perform a temporal artery biopsy on patients with PMR. It has been estimated that up to 50% of patients with PMR may have histological evidence of GCA. Further, the low doses of corticosteroids used to treat PMR will not prevent the complications of GCA. Many clinicians caring for patients with PMR and GCA do not recommend a biopsy if patients do not have symptoms or signs of GCA. If symptoms suggestive of GCA do develop, such as headache or scalp tenderness, a diagnostic biopsy can be performed.

Management

Patients with PMR can be readily treated with doses of prednisone of 10 to 20 mg/d. Symptoms respond and completely resolve promptly. Generally

TABLE 11.1 — 1990 CRITERIA FOR THE CLASSIFICATION OF GIANT CELL (TEMPORAL) ARTERITIS*

Criterion	Definition
Age at disease onset ≥ 50 years	Development of symptoms or findings beginning at age 50 or older
New headache	New onset of or new type of localized pain in the head
Temporal artery abnormality	Temporal artery tenderness to palpation or decreased pulsation, unrelated to arteriosclerosis of cervical arteries
Elevated erythrocyte sedimentation rate	Erythrocyte sedimentation rate ≥ 50 mm/h by the Westergren method
Abnormal artery biopsy	Biopsy specimen with artery showing vasculitis characterized by a predominance of mononuclear cell infiltration or granulomatous inflammation, usually with multinucleated giant cells

* For purposes of classification, a patient shall be said to have giant cell (temporal) arteritis if at least three of these five criteria are present. The presence of any three or more criteria yields a sensitivity of 93.5% and a specificity of 91.2%.

Hunder GG, et al. *Arthritis Rheum.* 1990;33:1122-1128.

after 1 to 2 weeks at these doses, the steroids can be tapered over several weeks to about 10 mg/d. Thereafter, tapering is guided by clinical response, recognizing that there may be discordance between symptoms and the ESR. Recurrence of symptoms with tapering may require dose increments to again control the disease; however, doses higher than those used initially to control the disease are not necessary.

When patients with PMR develop symptoms suggestive of GCA, higher doses of prednisone are administered while a temporal artery biopsy is arranged. Steroids over a week or two will not completely obscure the histological changes.

In an older patient where there is a high suspicion for GCA, high doses of corticosteroids (about 60 mg of prednisone) are administered while a confirmatory biopsy is performed. Once the diagnosis has been confirmed, steroids are continued until symptoms resolve and the ESR has normalized. This usually occurs within a month of starting treatment. Steroids can be tapered, guided by the recurrence of symptoms attributable to GCA and the ESR. Often the dose of prednisone can be tapered to about 20 mg/d within 2 or 3 months. Once that dose is reached, further steroid tapering is generally accomplished more slowly, but about 50% will be able to have their steroids discontinued within 2 years of starting therapy.

As always, the risk of iatrogenic hypercortisolism needs to be weighed against the concerns of disease progression. Patients who cannot have their steroids tapered below an acceptable point (often 20 mg of prednisone or less) may be candidates for other medications. Methotrexate and azathioprine have been used as steroid-sparing agents. In the case of methotrexate, the dose required may be relatively high (ie, 20 to 30 mg given as weekly pulses) in order to control the disease. In some patients, prolonged low-dose

147

steroids may be needed. Throughout the treatment course, efforts to limit calcium loss from bone should be instituted.

SUGGESTED READING

De Silva M, Hazleman BL. Azathioprine in giant cell arteritis/ polymyalgia rheumatica: a double-blind study. *Ann Rheum Dis.* 1986;45:136-138.

Fauchald P, Rygvold O, Oystese B. Temporal arteritis and polymyalgia rheumatica. Clinical and biopsy findings. *Ann Intern Med.* 1972;77:845-852.

Ferraccioli G, Salaffi F, De Vita S, Casatta L, Bartoli E. Methotrexate in polymyalgia rheumatica: preliminary results of an open, randomized study. *J Rheumatol.* 1996;23:624-628.

Hunder GG, Bloch DA, Michel BA, et al. The American College of Rheumatology 1990 criteria for the classification of giant cell arteritis. *Arthritis Rheum.* 1990;33:1122-1128.

12   Psoriatic Arthritis

The association between the skin disease psoriasis and arthritis has been recognized for nearly 200 years. For much of this time, the disorder was considered a coincidental occurrence of rheumatoid arthritis and psoriasis. With the discovery of rheumatoid factor, classification of psoriatic arthritis as a distinct disorder became possible.

Pathogenesis

The causes of both psoriasis and the associated arthritis are not known. The striking increased risk to first-degree relatives and the remarkable concordance in monozygotic twins (about 70%) provide evidence of a genetic association with this disorder. However, specific markers have not been found for most patients with psoriatic arthritis. Patients with psoriasis and axial skeletal disease do show an association with human leukocyte antigen (HLA)-B27.

Keratinocytes from patients with psoriatic arthritis divide more rapidly than normal and are more likely to express HLA-DR. Interaction with CD8$^+$ T cells is likely important. CD8$^+$ cells accumulate at inflammatory sites which, coupled with the observation that patients with human immunodeficiency virus (HIV) (and associated depletion of CD4$^+$ T cells) develop severe psoriasis, suggest a role for CD8$^+$ cells in the pathogenesis of this disease.

Occurrence

Approximately 0.1% of the population in the United States has psoriasis; of these, about 10% have concurrent arthritis. Psoriasis appears to be more common in whites and fairly unusual in Asians. Overall, women and men are at equal risk of developing psoriatic arthritis; however, women are more likely to develop a symmetrical arthritis and men a spondylitis. Onset of psoriasis occurs typically in the teens and twenties; the arthritis usually is seen a decade or two later.

Clinical Features

As noted above, in about 70% of cases, psoriasis develops prior to the arthritis. Ten percent of patients will develop arthritis at the same time they develop the skin rash. In the remainder, the arthritis precedes the onset of psoriasis. The arthritis associated with psoriasis is usually described as one of five specific clinical syndromes:
- Oligoarthritis (Figure 12.1)
- Axial involvement (Figure 12.2)
- Symmetrical polyarthritis (Figure 12.3)
- Distal involvement (Figure 12.4)
- Arthritis mutilans (Figure 12.5).

Oligoarthritis is the most common presentation of psoriatic arthritis and represents about 50% of the patients. Scattered small joints such as the proximal interphalangeal (PIP), distal interphalangeal (DIP), metatarsophalangeal, and metacarpophalangeal joints may be involved in association with a large joint such as the knee. The digit may be diffusely swollen, a "sausage" digit due to inflammation of the joint capsule and estheses.

Axial involvement represents about one third of the cases of psoriatic arthritis and is seen more often in males. It generally occurs many years after the psoriasis is present. Spondylitis or sacroiliitis may occur together or alone. In contrast to ankylosing spon-

FIGURE 12.1 — DIAGRAM DEPICTING AN OLIGOARTHRITIC DISTRIBUTION IN PSORIATIC ARTHRITIS

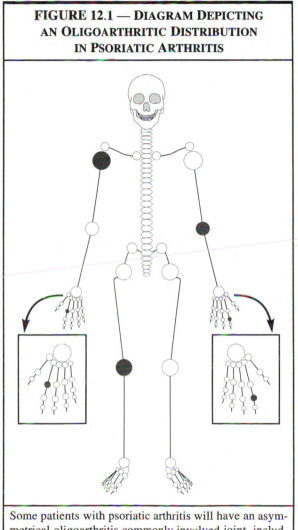

Some patients with psoriatic arthritis will have an asymmetrical oligoarthritis commonly involved joint, including the knee, shoulder, and scattered small joints in the hand.

12

FIGURE 12.2 — DIAGRAM DEPICTING JOINT INVOLVEMENT IN AXIAL ARTHRITIS

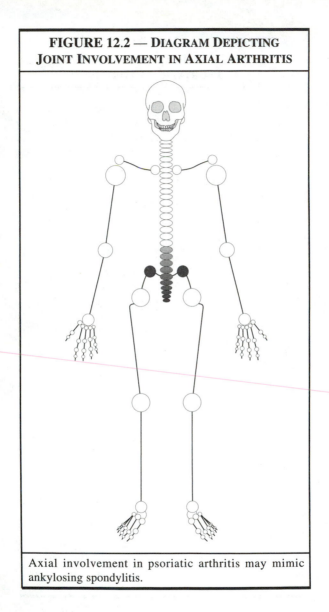

Axial involvement in psoriatic arthritis may mimic ankylosing spondylitis.

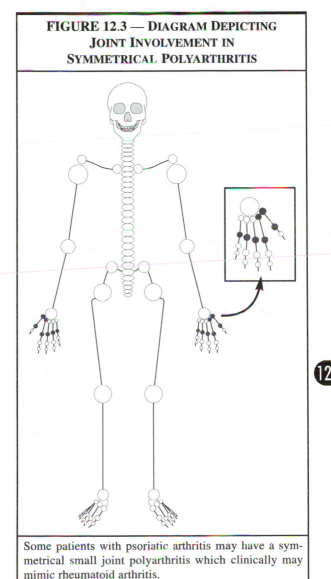

FIGURE 12.3 — DIAGRAM DEPICTING JOINT INVOLVEMENT IN SYMMETRICAL POLYARTHRITIS

Some patients with psoriatic arthritis may have a symmetrical small joint polyarthritis which clinically may mimic rheumatoid arthritis.

FIGURE 12.4 — DIAGRAM DEPICTING JOINT INVOLVEMENT IN ISOLATED DISTAL ARTHRITIS

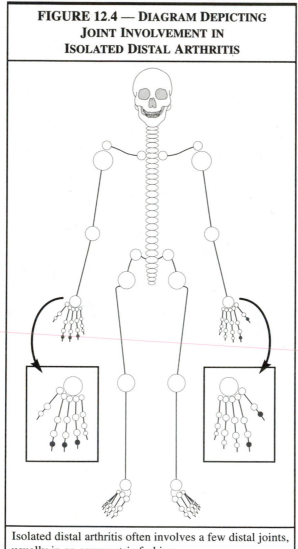

Isolated distal arthritis often involves a few distal joints, usually in an asymmetric fashion.

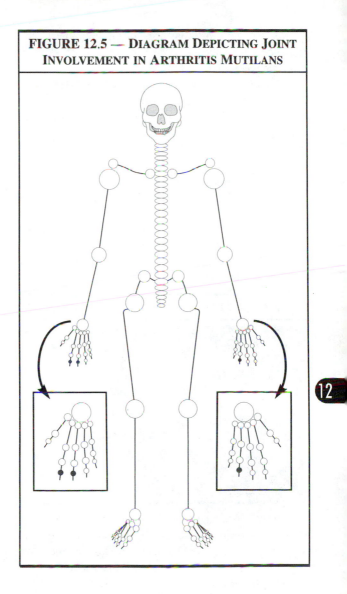

FIGURE 12.5 — DIAGRAM DEPICTING JOINT INVOLVEMENT IN ARTHRITIS MUTILANS

dylitis, the sacroiliitis is more often asymmetric and the spondylitis occurs more randomly, with skip lesions between involved sites.

A *symmetrical polyarthritis* is seen in at least 30% of patients with psoriatic arthritis and may evolve in an additive fashion from the oligoarticular form. In some patients, the joint distribution may be indistinguishable from rheumatoid arthritis. However, DIP joint involvement and a tendency to ankylose the joint are more common in psoriatic arthritis.

Isolated *DIP involvement* is seen in about 10% of patients with psoriatic arthritis. *Arthritis mutilans* is fortunately a rare presentation with resorption and telescoping of the involved phalanx (Figure 12.6). The fingers are most often involved, but similar changes can be found in the feet.

FIGURE 12.6 — ARTHRITIS MUTILANS

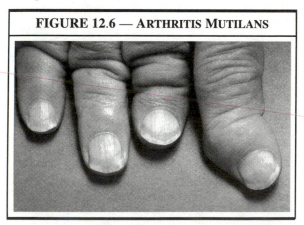

Extra-articular features characterize this disease. Indeed, it would be impossible to make the diagnosis without observing the characteristic skin changes. As noted, most patients will have skin disease at the time the arthritis appears. In those who do not, the diagnosis may be considered based upon the articular presentation but cannot be confirmed until the rash appears. Most patients with psoriatic arthritis will have psoriasis vulgaris, but occasionally a patient will present with erythrodermic or pustular forms (Figure 12.7). The typical lesion is a well demarcated, hyperkeratotic, erythematous plaque with a silvery scale. The lesions vary from the 1 mm guttate lesions to larger plaques spanning several centimeters. Lesions may be found nearly anywhere on the body, but have a predilection for the scalp and the extensor surfaces of the elbows and knees. Careful and complete skin examinations may reveal psoriatic plaques in the umbilicus, scalp, or perineum which may add in confirming the diagnosis. There is no correlation between the extent or severity of the skin disease and the articular findings.

Nail involvement is typical of psoriatic arthritis and can be useful in making the diagnosis where the

---

FIGURE 12.7 — TYPICAL SKIN CHANGES OF PSORIASIS

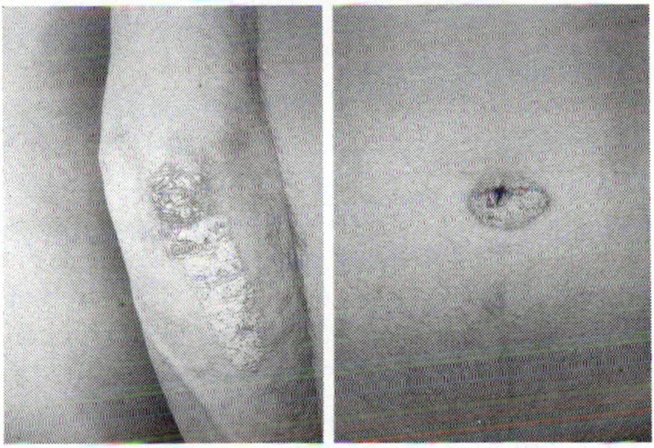

Typical scaly, hyperkeratotic lesions seen in patients with psoriasis. Extent and severity of the skin lesions do not correlate with the arthritis. Lesions may be small and located in areas such as the scalp, umbilicus or anus where they may escape detection and not be looked for specifically.

arthritis is otherwise unexplained (Figure 12.8). About two thirds of patients with psoriatic arthritis will have nail pits; twice as likely as those with psoriasis alone. Normal individuals may have a few pits per nail, but it has been suggested that patients with psoriatic arthritis will have more than 20 pits per nail. Onycholysis, nail fragility, and ridging are other more nonspecific nail findings in psoriatic arthritis.

FIGURE 12.8 — NAIL INVOLVEMENT TYPICAL OF PSORIATIC ARTHRITIS

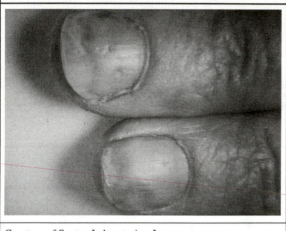

Courtesy of Syntex Laboratories, Inc.

Other extra-articular features seen in patients with psoriatic arthritis include conjunctivitis and, rarely, iritis or episcleritis. Eye findings may be more common in those with axial skeleton disease. Aortic and cardiac conduction abnormalities are unusual in psoriatic arthritis.

Diagnosis

The diagnosis of psoriatic arthritis is easily made in the presence of an inflammatory arthropathy and psoriasis. Occasional confusion occurs when a patient

158

with known psoriasis develops osteoarthritis. This is particularly true when there is involvement of the DIP and PIP joints. In other situations, seborrhea or eczema may be confused with psoriasis. If psoriatic skin changes are not apparent, the differential becomes even broader. Other disorders such as Reiter's syndrome and ankylosing spondylitis may be difficult to differentiate. In older individuals, a diffusely swollen toe may be confused with gout.

Laboratory Tests and Radiographs

There are no specific laboratory tests for psoriatic arthritis. Acute phase reactants such as erythrocyte sedimentation rate and C-reactive protein may be elevated. Rheumatoid factor is usually negative. Patients who have extensive psoriasis may have increased uric acid levels.

Radiographs of involved joints will often reveal marginal erosions, but often without the osteopenia more characteristic of rheumatoid arthritis. The distribution of changes may help clarify the diagnosis. Distal involvement in the hands and acro-osteolysis (erosion of the terminal tuft of the distal phalanx) are sometimes seen in psoriatic arthritis patients (Figure 12.9). Similarly, so is sacroiliitis and spondylitis. Isolated destruction of an individual joint, in particular the "pencil in cup" deformity, may be suggestive of psoriatic arthritis.

Management

In comparison to rheumatoid arthritis, this arthritis is more readily controlled and is less likely to lead to disability. Most medications which are used to treat the arthritis do not affect the skin disease and vice versa. Often, the skin disease can be treated with topical agents. Topical steroids and topical derivatives of

FIGURE 12.9 — DISTAL INVOLVEMENT IN THE HANDS AND ACRO-OSTEOLYSIS OF PSORIATIC ARTHRITIS

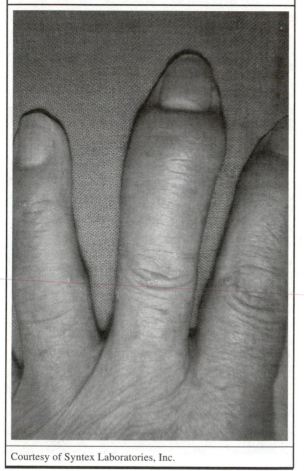

Courtesy of Syntex Laboratories, Inc.

vitamin D are both effective in treating the skin disease. In more resistant cases, pulsed ultraviolet actinotherapy is effective.

Nonsteroidal anti-inflammatory drugs are the mainstay of therapy for the articular disease in most patients. As with other forms of arthritis, if a small number of joints are not controlled, intra-articular steroids may be useful. Care must be taken to not inject through psoriasiform skin as this may lead to bacterial seeding of the joint.

In those patients whose disease is still not controlled, a number of slow-acting agents have been found to be effective. Included among this group are the antimalarials, gold salts, sulfasalazine, 6-mercaptopurine, and methotrexate. There is no convincing evidence that gold salts, antimalarials, or sulfasalazine will control the skin disease. In contrast, methotrexate is useful in treating both the skin and articular disease. Concerns have been raised about liver toxicity of methotrexate in patients with psoriasis; however, repeat liver biopsies in small numbers of patients have not shown progression of changes seen in the baseline biopsies. Other agents, including colchicine and cyclosporin A, have been shown in short-term studies to be effective.

SUGGESTED READING

Baker H. Epidemiological aspects of psoriasis and arthritis. *Br J Dermatol*. 1966;78:249-262.

Clegg DO, Reda DJ, Mejias E, et al. Comparison of sulfasalazine and placebo in the treatment of psoriatic arthritis. A Department of Veterans Affairs Cooperative Study. *Arthritis Rheum*. 1996; 39:2013-2020.

Cuéllar ML, Silveira LH, Espinoza LR. Recent developments in psoriatic arthritis. *Curr Opin Rheumatol*. 1994;6:378-383.

Espinoza LR, Zakraoui L, Espinoza CG, et al. Psoriatic arthritis: clinical response and side effects to methotrexate therapy. *J Rheumatol*. 1992;19:872-879.

13 Reiter's Syndrome

Reiter's syndrome is considered one of the seronegative spondyloarthropathies (SNSAs) and includes a peripheral arthritis with characteristic extra-articular features. Although similar clinical descriptions had previously appeared, Hans Reiter's description in 1916 of a Prussian lieutenant who developed arthritis, conjunctivitis, and urethritis after an infectious diarrheal illness led to the eponym. Recognition that several organisms are associated with the development of a complete or incomplete Reiter's syndrome led to its designation as a reactive arthritis, although both terms are frequently used interchangeably.

Pathogenesis

As with the other SNSAs, the specific processes leading to the clinical manifestations of this disorder are not known. Overall, the association between Reiter's and human leukocyte antigen (HLA)-B27 is strong, with at least half of patients having this marker. However, over 90% of those with Reiter's syndrome and spondylitis will be HLA-B27–positive. In ethnic groups where HLA-B27 is rare, so is Reiter's syndrome; however, the converse is not necessarily so. In two American Indian groups, the Haida and Pima Indians, expression of HLA-B27 (and ankylosing spondylitis [AS]) is common, but Reiter's syndrome is not often found.

Since 1916, it has been recognized that a number of infectious illnesses appear to trigger the development of this arthritis. Organisms which have been associated with reactive arthritis include:

- Enteric:
  - *Salmonella enteritidis*, *S parathyphia*, and *S typhimurium*
  - *Shigella flexneri*
  - *Camplyobacter fetus* and *C jejuni*
  - *Yersinia enterocolitica* and *Y pseudotuberculosis*
  - *Clostridium difficile*
- Venereal infections:
  - *Chlamydia pneumoniae* and *C trachomatis*
  - *Ureaplasma urealyticum.*

Interestingly, immunohistochemical and *in situ* hybridization studies have demonstrated that antigenic and nuclear material from some of these organisms is detectable in synovium from patients with Reiter's syndrome, but viable organisms are not. The connection between these infectious organisms and HLA-B27 cannot totally account for the disease because in epidemic infections, only about 20% of HLA-B27–positive individuals develop Reiter's syndrome.

The relationship between human immunodeficiency virus (HIV) infection and reactive arthritis remains uncertain. Some authors have suggested a relationship, but HIV-positive patients do not seem to develop reactive arthritis any more often when other risk factors are controlled.

Occurrence

The prevalence of Reiter's syndrome is largely unknown. To some extent this is due to:
- A lack of a consistent set of diagnostic criteria
- The potential stigma of reporting venereal-associated disorders
- The difficulty recognizing asymptomatic infections

- The younger age group most often afflicted with this disorder.

However, in perhaps the most extensive survey, which was undertaken between 1950 and 1980, the age-adjusted incidence of Reiter's syndrome in men was 3.5 cases per 100,000 population. In more recent work from Scandinavia, the incidence of reactive arthritis associated with chlamydiae was nearly 5 cases per 100,000. Studies of epidemic dysentery have suggested that, overall, about 5% of infected individuals will develop arthritis; but, as noted above, 20% of those who are HLA-B27–positive may develop arthritis. Incidence of *C trachomatis*-related reactive arthritis is slightly less, with up to 3% of infected individuals developing chronic arthritis.

As might be expected, this is a disorder of the younger adult. Some reports indicate that over 95% of those with reactive arthritis are males. However, this is probably an overestimate reflecting the sometimes absent or subtle clinical signs of urethritis in women. Nonetheless, reactive arthritis is still predominantly a male disorder.

Clinical Features

In those individuals who have had a recognizable infectious illness as the presumed precipitant of reactive arthritis, symptoms tend to start about 3 or 4 weeks after the infectious event. In those who have had an infectious diarrheal illness, the gastrointestinal symptoms will most often have resolved by the time arthritis develops. However, roughly two thirds of those who are thought to have reactive arthritis will not have a clinically defined precipitating event. The arthritis is best described as a predominantly lower extremity asymmetric oligoarthritis (Figure 13.1).

FIGURE 13.1 — DIAGRAM DEPICTING JOINT INVOLVEMENT IN REITER'S SYNDROME

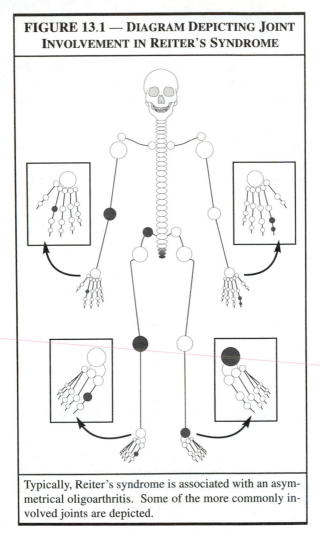

Typically, Reiter's syndrome is associated with an asymmetrical oligoarthritis. Some of the more commonly involved joints are depicted.

Onset is usually abrupt and joints are swollen and often erythematous. In some patients, there is accompanying fever, raising the specter of a septic arthritis. Nearly half will have only lower-extremity involvement, and the knee is the most commonly involved joint. The small joints of the hands and/or feet may be involved and the digit may appear to be diffusely swollen: the so-called "sausage" digit. The diffuse swelling or dactylitis is secondary to inflammation of the joint and periarticular structures. A rare patient may have a symmetrical polyarthritis which, based only on joint distribution, may be difficult to differentiate from rheumatoid arthritis.

For most individuals, the arthritis resolves in about 12 months, but many will continue to have musculoskeletal complaints long after this time. Between 10% and 20% of patients with reactive arthritis will develop a chronic arthritis that is usually relapsing and remitting in character. Symptoms suggesting axial skeletal involvement are present in over one half of patients with reactive arthritis, but fewer than 25% will have radiographic evidence of sacroiliitis. The axial involvement in reactive arthritis at times can be differentiated from AS by asymmetry of the sacroiliac (SI) joint involvement and the presence of skip lesions in the remainder of the axial skeleton.

Enthesopathy is common in reactive arthritis and involvement of tendon and ligamental insertion sites around the foot are most frequently noted. Other enthesopathic involvement is commonly around the pelvis and chest wall.

Extra-articular features of the disease are important in its characterization. Genitourinary inflammation occurs in about one third of patients. Typically symptoms (including a sterile purulent discharge) are seen early in the course and are seen even in patients who have had a dysenteric illness. In women, the symptoms may be subtle or attributed to other processes. Painless oral ulceration may be found on the tongue or palate. Circinate balanitis, a shallow ulcer on the glans or penile shaft, is found in about 20% of patients (Figure 13.2). Keratoderma blennorrhagica is a pustular lesion found in about a quarter of patients

FIGURE 13.2 — CIRCINATE BALANITIS

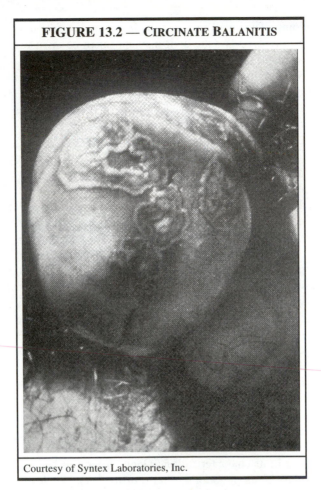

Courtesy of Syntex Laboratories, Inc.

with Reiter's syndrome (Figure 13.3). This lesion is histologically indistinguishable from pustular psoriasis and is usually found on the soles of the feet or the palms of the hands. Nails are frequently found to be thickened and raised, but do not have the excess pits seen with psoriasis.

Ocular manifestations, in particular conjunctivitis, represent one of the classic Reiter's triad of symptoms. Conjunctivitis is manifest by pain and injec-

**FIGURE 13.3 — REITER'S SYNDROME:
TYPICAL SKIN AND NAIL CHANGES**

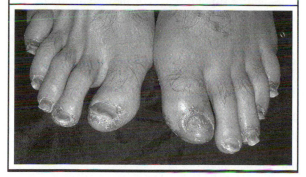

tion and is often seen early in the course and may re-cur episodically. Anterior uveitis presents acutely and may be observed even late in the course. Even with treatment, chronic uveitis can lead to visual impairment.

Aortitis and cardiac conduction system defects occur in a rare patient who has long-standing arthritis.

Finally, systemic complaints can be burdensome. Fever may be present and be of a degree to suggest a septic process. This may be accompanied by anorexia, weight loss, and fatigue.

13

Diagnosis

The diagnosis of reactive arthritis is considered in an individual who has an asymmetric oligoarthritis and typical extra-articular features. The most difficult disorders to differentiate are other SNSAs. Early in the course, it is important to exclude septic arthritis. Crystal-induced arthritis may be a consideration, particularly in an older individual.

Arthritis also has been reported in association with several inflammatory cutaneous disorders. Peripheral and a somewhat distinctive axial arthritis have been reported in patients with acne conglobate or hidradenitis suppurativa. In these individuals, the axial involvement predominates in the anterior chest wall and tends to spare the SI joints.

Laboratory Tests and Radiographs

Laboratory tests performed on patients with reactive arthritis are reflective of the systemic inflammation. Acute phase proteins are generally elevated as are white blood cell counts and platelets. Patients may have anemia of chronic disease.

Synovial fluid is inflammatory in nature with elevated neutrophil counts. Occasionally a "Reiter's cell" will be observed, which is a large mononuclear phagocyte that has ingested several neutrophils.

Radiographic findings in patients with reactive arthritis are similar to those seen in other SNSAs. Periosteal reaction is seen at sites of enthesopathy, particularly of the Achilles tendon (Figure 13.4). Marginal erosions may be seen in involved joints. Axial skeletal disease may be just like that seen in patients with AS, but patients with reactive arthritis may have asymmetrical changes in the SI joints and skip lesions in the remainder of the axial skeleton.

Management

Most patients with Reiter's syndrome can be managed with nonsteroidal anti-inflammatory drugs (NSAIDs). Typically, use of anti-inflammatory doses of these medications can:
- Reduce stiffness
- Reduce swelling
- Alleviate pain
- Promote range of motion.

FIGURE 13.4 — REITER'S SYNDROME:
ENTHESOPATHY

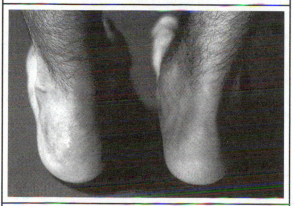

Enthesopathic changes (inflammation at insertion sites of tendons and ligaments) are common in Reiter's syndrome and other seronegative spondyloarthropathies.

Courtesy of the Arthritis Foundation.

When these drugs are coupled with strengthening and range of motion exercises, most patients can be adequately treated until their arthritis remits.

In patients whose chronic arthritis is not adequately controlled with this regimen, several alternative agents have been studied. Intra-articular corticosteroids are useful when the arthritis involving a small number of joints is not adequately controlled. There are few indications for systemic steroids. Alternatively, sulfasalazine, methotrexate, and azathioprine have been used successfully in treatment of patients with Reiter's syndrome who have not responded to NSAIDs. However, these drugs do not seem to affect the axial disease.

Since this disorder appears to be triggered by an infectious organism and, in some patients, evidence exists for persistence of the organism in the joint, the question of antibiotic therapy is often raised. It has

13

been recommended that the physician prescribe antibiotic therapy early in the course of the infection, particularly when an inciting organism can be identified. Patients with chlamydia-induced arthritis may have a shorter duration of disease and a less severe course when treated with tetracyclines for more than 3 months. Other studies of patients with postdysentery arthritis have failed to demonstrate any antibiotic efficacy. Based on available studies, it would be difficult to recommend a prolonged course of antibiotics in a patient with Reiter's syndrome.

SUGGESTED READING

Arnett FC. Seronegative spondyloarthropathies. *Bull Rheum Dis.* 1987;37:1-12.

Clegg DO, Reda DJ, Weisman MH, et al. Comparison of sulfasalazine and placebo in the treatment of reactive arthritis (Reiter's Syndrome). *Arthritis Rheum.* 1996;39:2021-2027.

Creemers MC, van Riel RL, Franssen MJ, van de Putte LB, Gribnau FW. Second-line therapy in seronegative spondylarthropathies. *Semin Arthritis Rheum.* 1994;24:71-81.

Keat A, Rowe I. Reiter's syndrome and associated arthritides. *Rheum Dis Clin North Am.* 1991;17:25-42.

Taurog JD, Richardson JA, Croft JT, et al. The germfree state prevents development of gut and joint inflammatory disease in HLA-B27 transgenic rats. *J Exp Med.* 1994;180:2359-2364.

14 Rheumatoid Arthritis

A significant amount has been learned about the mechanisms responsible for tissue injury in rheumatoid arthritis (RA), one of the most common forms of inflammatory arthritis. Much of this knowledge is being applied and new therapies are being developed, which should interdict the process.

Pathogenesis

The cartilage damage that occurs in patients with RA is due to at least three processes:

- Cells in synovial fluid, predominantly neutrophils, are activated and appear to degrade the surface layer of the articular cartilage.
- Chondrocytes, influenced by cytokines such as interleukin (IL)-1 and tumor necrosis factor (TNF)-α, digest surrounding cartilage.
- Most importantly, the synovium (composed of cells of macrophage and fibroblast origin) directly digests subjacent cartilage and releases a variety of inflammatory molecules including TNF-α and IL-1 (which not only influence other cells, but are responsible for some of the systemic effects of this disease).

The actual mechanisms responsible for initiating RA have not been elucidated. Persons carrying the class II human leukocyte antigen (HLA)-DR4 have a risk factor for the development of RA. This, coupled with the observation that family members are at higher risk of developing RA, has led to the hypothesis that it is a polygenic disease.

The subsequent observation that a five-amino-acid sequence in the third hypervariable region (rheumatoid epitome) was linked to the development of RA intensified these arguments. However, the universal importance of this sequence has recently been questioned, as studies in other groups, including black Americans, did not find the same correlation. Others have suggested that the primary lesion may be in the synovial fibroblast which, in culture, divides more rapidly and is more resistant to senescence than normal fibroblasts.

Occurrence

Rheumatoid arthritis occurs worldwide, in all populations and ethnic groups. By definition, it is seen in individuals over 16 years of age (although an identical disease is seen in some younger children), and the prevalence of the disease increases with age. Women tend to get this disease about 2 to 3 times as often as men. RA is common and about 1% of the population has the disease. There are a few groups in which the prevalence is increased, such as certain groups of American Indians, where as many as 5% may have the disease.

Clinical Features

In most patients, the clinical picture is dominated by the articular features of the disease. Generally the disease onset is rather insidious, with symptoms developing over several weeks or months. Occasionally, patients will have an explosive onset or an intermittent palindromic onset. Morning stiffness, a hallmark of inflammatory arthritis, is prominent and may last hours or all day. The extent of morning stiffness correlates with overall disease activity and resolves when the disease is in remission.

Rheumatoid arthritis is a symmetrical polyarthritis. Commonly involved joints are the:

- Small joints of the hands and feet
- Wrists
- Metacarpophalangeals (MCPs)
- Metatarsophalangeals.

However, as shown in Table 14.1, large joints are frequently involved. Joint pain is often described as tenderness or aching pain and stiffness, which is felt diffusely throughout the joint. Interestingly, as demonstrated by O'Sullivan and Cathcart, as many as half of patients who may be initially diagnosed as having RA will no longer be similarly considered 2 years later. In contrast, most patients with established RA will have a progressive course, and it is rare for them to enter a remission. In some studies, as many as 50% of patients will have disability from work within 5 years of disease onset.

Over time deformities develop, including volar subluxation of the carpal bone, ulnar drift of the MCPs, and swan neck or boutonnière deformity (Figure 14.1). Functional limitations range from clumsiness in fine motor activities to inability to perform many of the activities of daily living, including dressing and eating. In addition to the hand deformities, synovium may compress the median or, less often, the ulnar nerve (at the wrist or elbow), and weakness and muscle atrophy may develop.

Elbow involvement is frequently seen and easily demonstrated on physical examination. As synovial fluid accumulates in the elbow, pressure rises and the natural tendency is to flex the joint (similar observations may be made for the knee and hip) to increase the volume and lower pressure, thereby decreasing symptoms. Unfortunately, this may rapidly lead to the development of flexion contracture.

14

TABLE 14.1 — JOINTS INVOLVED IN RHEUMATOID ARTHRITIS*

Joint Involved	Percent Initially Involved			Percent Ultimately Involved
	Right	Left	Bilateral	
Shoulder	37	42	30	47
Knee	35	30	24	56
Ankle	25	23	18	53
Elbow	20	15	14	21
Wrist	60	57	48	82
Metacarpophalangeal	65	58	52	87
Proximal interphalangeal	63	53	45	63
Metatarsophalangeal	48	47	43	48

* Other joints (eg, distal interphalangeal joints) are not tabulated here.

Adapted from: Harris ED Jr. In: *Textbook of Rheumatology*. Vol 1. 4th ed. 1981:932.

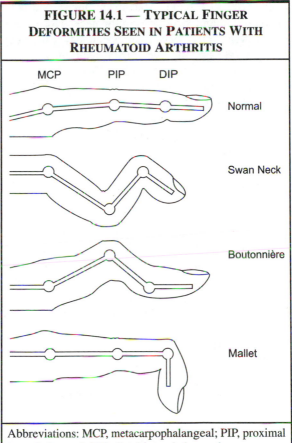

FIGURE 14.1 — TYPICAL FINGER DEFORMITIES SEEN IN PATIENTS WITH RHEUMATOID ARTHRITIS

MCP PIP DIP

Normal

Swan Neck

Boutonnière

Mallet

Abbreviations: MCP, metacarpophalangeal; PIP, proximal interphalangeal; DIP, distal interphalangeal.

Shoulder involvement is generally seen as a decrease in abduction or rotation, particularly when motion in other joints allows for the patient to raise the hand over the head. The rotator cuff may become attenuated and rupture, further limiting joint motion.

Cervical spine involvement may precipitate one of the few emergencies associated with caring for patients with RA. Generally, the involvement is high in the cervical spine. Dissolution of the odontoid or lateral masses of C1 may lead to instability and compression of major structures in the neck. Cord, nerve root, or vertebral artery compression may lead to dizziness, weakness, and even visual symptoms.

Hip disease in RA is common, but may be present with pain being the only indication. Symptoms are usually felt in the buttock or groin or may radiate to the knee. Limited rotation or the development of flexion contractures may be the earliest physical findings.

Knee involvement is usually tricompartmental and may be a major source of disability. Instability and contractures may develop, compounding the problem.

Foot involvement is fairly characteristic. Typically, there is eversion at the ankle, lengthening and flattening of the longitudinal arch, and cocking up of the toes. As this happens, the fat pad (which is usually under the metatarsal heads) subluxes, making ambulation on the metatarsal heads painful. Frequently, callosities develop and may even break down.

■ Extra-articular Features

Rheumatoid nodules are the most common extra-articular feature associated with RA. Generally, they are seen in patients who are rheumatoid factor positive and are frequently found on sites such as the olecranon, fingers, or other sites of pressure. Rarely, they may be found internally where their presence may interfere with function, eg, the cardiac conduction system or the meninges.

Eye problems are also frequently seen and, in most cases, are manifest by dry eyes and/or mouth or erythema due to episcleritis. In most situations, attributing sicca complaints to RA or to the myriad of other causes of dry mucosa is not important, since therapy is largely symptomatic. On the other hand, an occasional patient may develop scleritis, which is usually quite painful and may lead to thinning and rupture of the globe and blindness.

Skin ulcers are seen in patients with severe progressive RA. Generally, multiple factors may contribute to their developing, including poor nutrition, edema, skin thinning due to steroids, and even small vessel vasculitis. Rarely, larger or visceral vessels may be involved (Figure 14.2), which can lead to digital ischemia or mononeuritis multiplex.

Rheumatoid arthritis can involve the lung in several ways. Most commonly, interstitial fibrotic pictures may be seen on chest radiographs. Changes are generally noted in the lung bases. Patients, limited in mobility due to their articular disease, may not even be aware of the pulmonary involvement. Some may simply have a dry, nonproductive cough. Pulmonary nodules, which may cavitate, are an occasional finding on chest radiographs. Histologically, they are identical to rheumatoid nodules found elsewhere. Usually, they are not associated with symptoms, but differentiation from metastatic disease or an infection may be difficult without a biopsy. Pulmonary effusions are not uncommon, but rarely are clinically significant. When large enough to be sampled, they are characteristically effusions, often have decreased glucose concentrations, and may be frankly purulent. A rare patient may have pulmonary vasculitis and symptoms of pulmonary hypertension.

Felty's syndrome is defined clinically as the neutropenia and splenomegaly occurring in a patient with RA. The causes of the neutropenia are heterogeneous, including decreased marrow production and peripheral destruction. Recently, it has been recognized that some patients who have expansion in the marrow of cells that are phenotypically large granular lymphocytes may also have neutropenia.

14

FIGURE 14.2 — VASCULITIC LESIONS IN RHEUMATOID ARTHRITIS

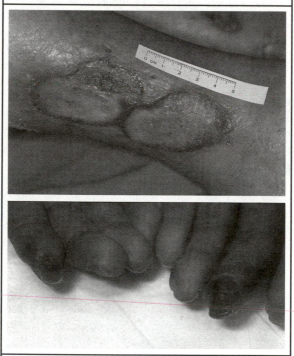

Top: Leg ulcers due to vasculitis from rheumatoid arthritis. Often the ulcers are also complicated by factors including arterial and venous insufficiency. *Bottom*: Ischemic changes in the fingers due to digital artery vasculitis.

Other conditions, such as myositis, pericardial effusions, and development of amyloidosis, are rarely seen in patients with RA.

Laboratory Features and Radiographs

There is no laboratory test which is specific for RA. Rheumatoid factor, as generally measured, is composed of immunoglobulin M (IgM) molecules that bind to the Fc portion of IgG. About 5% to 10% of normal individuals may have rheumatoid factors detectable in their serum by standard laboratory testing. More sensitive tests can detect them in nearly everyone. Nearly 85% of patients with RA will have rheumatoid factor detectable by routine testing in their serum, but only about half may have it detectable at the time of symptom onset. Although patients with more severe disease are likely to have a higher titer of rheumatoid factor, there is considerable overlap and there is no evidence that it changes as a measure of disease activity. Antinuclear antibodies are frequently seen in the serum of patients with RA and do not necessarily reflect an overlap syndrome.

Other laboratory tests that may be abnormal in RA generally reflect the fact that it is a chronic systemic rheumatic disease. Most patients with RA will have anemia of chronic disease. This may be further exacerbated by blood loss associated with medication use. Typically, red cells are either normocytic or microcytic. Reticulocyte counts are decreased and response to exogenous erythropoietin is diminished. Platelet counts are usually elevated, as are white blood cell (WBC) counts. WBC counts may be diminished due to Felty's syndrome, iatrogenic causes, or intercurrent illnesses.

Erythrocyte sedimentation rates and C-reactive protein (CRP) are usually elevated in patients with RA. Both of these are used as measures of disease activity within an individual patient, but there is considerable variability among patients.

Early in the course, plain radiographs simply demonstrate periarticular osteoporosis and soft-tissue swelling. Marginal erosions appear later at the cartilage pannus junction. As the disease progresses, joint space is lost and deformities develop. Diagnostically, radiographs of the hands and feet are most useful.

Diagnosis

Frequently, the diagnosis of RA can be made based on the initial history and physical examination. A patient with a symmetrical, predominantly small-joint, inflammatory polyarthritis will often have RA. Diagnostic criteria have been developed and are shown in Table 14.2. In such a patient, the finding that rheumatoid factor is present in the serum is reassuring but should not be relied on in the face of negative findings on examination. Occasionally, patients with gout, pseudogout or even lupus may present with similar findings, and either extra-articular features or synovial fluid examination may be helpful.

TABLE 14.2 — AMERICAN RHEUMATISM ASSOCIATION 1987 CRITERIA

- Morning stiffness > 1 h
- Swelling of three or more joints for > 6 wks
- Arthritis of hand joints > 6 wks
- Symmetrical joint swelling
- Nodules
- Rheumatoid factor
- Typical radiographic changes of rheumatoid arthritis

Arnett FC, et al. *Arthritis Rheum.* 1988;31:315-324.

Management

Prior to embarking on a discussion of pharmacologic therapies, it is useful to remember that a number of other interventions are important in the management of this chronic disease. Education, particularly early in the course, can frequently allay fears and correct misconceptions. Exercise maintains strength and range of motion and may limit the development of osteoporosis. Rest of an involved joint also is appropriate at times during the meandering course of RA.

Pharmacological Therapy

Presently available pharmacological therapy of RA generally involves three types of drugs:

- Nonsteroidal anti-inflammatory drugs (NSAIDs)
- Corticosteroids
- Slow-acting, antirheumatic agents.

■ Nonsteroidal Anti-inflammatory Drugs

The NSAIDs were once thought to be the primary agents necessary for treatment of early RA. Recognition of their side effects and limited efficacy have led to a reassessment of their position.

The oldest NSAID is aspirin. It is inexpensive, but toxicity and its peculiar pharmacokinetics have limited its use. In anti-inflammatory doses, there usually is saturation of certain metabolic pathways, and slight increases in dose can lead to significant increases in drug blood levels. In most individuals, toxicity is heralded by tinnitus. However, in the elderly who have lost high-frequency auditory acuity, the first signs of toxicity may be confusion or other signs of a severe metabolic acidosis. Aspirin that is not enteric coated is associated with higher gastrointestinal (GI) blood loss than other NSAIDs.

Over the last 2 decades there has been a dramatic increase in the number of NSAIDs available to US physicians. When used in anti-inflammatory doses, each is effective in the treatment of RA. The toxicities and perhaps efficacy are linked to their inhibition of cyclooxygenase (COX), which thus limits production of certain prostaglandins. However, prostaglandins play an important protective role, particularly in the stomach and kidney. GI toxicity is reported in about 20% of patients taking NSAIDS and about 1% have significant GI toxicity as defined by perforations, ulcers or bleeding.

There is little information to suggest that there are significant differences between NSAIDS in terms of either efficacy or toxicity when used in equivalent anti-inflammatory doses. There are kinetic differences between these drugs which allow for differences in dosing regimens. NSAIDS that have long enough half-lives so that they can be given once or twice a day are associated with better compliance.

In terms of toxicity, there are a few differences among NSAIDs. Indomethacin appears to have a higher incidence of central nervous system side effects, which are generally manifest as confusion, often a problem in the older patient. It has been suggested that this is due to the fact that indomethacin is structurally similar to serotonin. Sulindac is reputed to be renal sparing. The rationale for this claim has been the fact that sulindac is a pro-drug activated in the liver. When it passes through the kidney, the drug is re-inactivated, leading to a hypothesis that it may be renal sparing. Nonetheless, there have been reports of renal failure which have implicated sulindac.

■ COX-2 Targeted NSAIDs

The first available COX-2 targeted agent, celecoxib, has been shown to be effective as naproxen and other NSAIDs in the treatment of RA. In a 12-week multicenter, placebo-controlled, double-blind trial involving 1149 RA patients, celecoxib produced a significant decrease in the number of tender/painful joints and of swollen joints in treated patients. The percentage of patients responding is shown in Figure 14.3. Celecoxib produced significant results in all dosage groups. The maximal effect of celecoxib was evident at 2 weeks and was sustained throughout the 12-week study.

Several studies have further demonstrated that GI tolerability of celecoxib is comparable to placebo and significantly better than naproxen. Endoscopic stud-

184

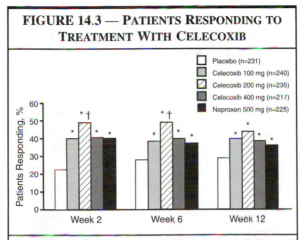

FIGURE 14.3 — PATIENTS RESPONDING TO TREATMENT WITH CELECOXIB

Patients classified as responders by American College of Rheumatology (ACR-20) criteria at 2, 6, and 12 weeks. Responders were defined as those with at least 20% improvement from baseline in the number of tender/painful joints and number of swollen joints, as well as at least 20% improvement in at least 3 of the following: (1) Physician's Global Assessment, (2) Patient's Global Assessment, (3) patients assessment of pain, (4) C-reactive protein levels, or (5) health assessment questionnaire functional disability score. All active treatments were statistically significantly superior to placebo ($P < 0.05$) at all 3 assessment times (asterisks). Dagger indicates significantly different from naproxen ($P < 0.05$) celecoxib and naproxen were both administered twice daily for all dosages.

Simon LS, et al. *JAMA.* 1999;282:1924.

ies have indicated that when patients with RA are treated with either celecoxib, naproxen, or placebo, those treated with celecoxib develop ulcers no more often than the placebo group and much less often than the naproxen-treated group (Figure 14.4). Since its introduction, there has been extensive experience with this medication and post-marketing surveys represent-

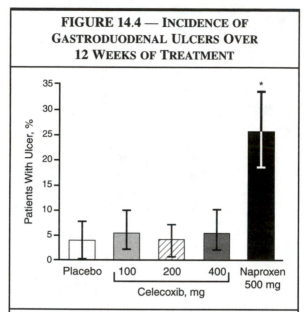

FIGURE 14.4 — INCIDENCE OF GASTRODUODENAL ULCERS OVER 12 WEEKS OF TREATMENT

An ulcer was defined as any break in the mucosa at least 3 mm in diameter with unequivocal depth. For each patient there were 3 possible outcomes; known ulcer, known no ulcer, and unknown. Any endoscopic finding other than ulcer was categorized as unknown if the data were obtained before the 12-week visit. Naproxen-treated patients had a significantly greater incidence of gastroduodenal ulcers than did patients treated with either celecoxib or placebo ($P < 0.001$). The incidences of gastroduodenal ulcers in the celecoxib treatment groups were similar to that in placebo-treated patients ($P > 0.40$). Error bars indicate 95% confidence intervals. Asterisk indicates $P < 0.001$ vs all other treatments. Celecoxib and naproxen were both administered twice daily for all dosages.

Simon LS, et al. *JAMA*. 1999;282:1926.

ing over 340,000 patient years of use remarkably suggest that the rate of significant GI complications with celecoxib (ie, ulcers, perforation, and bleeding) are very low and comparable to background rates.

■ Corticosteroids

Heralded as the cure for many inflammatory disorders, including RA, corticosteroids have had a checkered past. The apparent cures associated with high doses of corticosteroids were soon recognized to be hollow as patients began presenting with the signs and symptoms due to the ravages of iatrogenic hypercortisolism. In response, there was a period of time where steroids were not even considered for therapy of RA.

More recently, the role of corticosteroids has been reassessed and the utility of low-dose steroids has been recognized. Response to steroids is prompt, and recent evidence suggests that doses of prednisone under 10 mg/d may be effective in slowing radiographic disease progression. This observation is in keeping with findings demonstrating that steroids down-regulate production of inflammatory cytokines, collagenase and other degradative proteases.

Despite these observations, use of steroids in RA should be undertaken with care. Even low doses have distinct metabolic effects. It takes few patients with thinned purpuric skin, slumped over with osteoporosis, to reinforce the downside of long-term glucocorticoid use.

■ Slow-Acting Antirheumatic Drugs

Overall, compounds considered as slow-acting antirheumatic drugs (SAARDs) have few chemical similarities. In contrast to NSAIDS and corticosteroids, they are relatively slow acting. The clinically apparent onset of action may take weeks or even months, sometimes trying the patience of both physi-

187

cian and patient. These drugs have been generally evaluated in the face of ongoing therapy with NSAIDs and low-dose corticosteroids, and have been found to have additional benefit. Although there is little information indicating that these compounds regularly induce disease remission, it is believed that they slow disease progression. However, once cartilage integrity has been violated, there is limited opportunity for repair. Thus, there is some urgency to begin these compounds early in the course of the disease.

There are quite a number of SAARDs. To a large extent, the mechanisms of action of these agents is unknown. It is difficult to extrapolate results of short-term cell culture studies, often in the presence of drug levels which greatly exceed those found *in vivo*.

To a large extent, the order for use of SAARDs is a matter of choice. However, there has been a definite shift in the pattern of SAARD use over the last several years. Many rheumatologists no longer use compounds such as gold and penicillamine. Nonetheless, each drug has been shown to be effective in therapy of RA and may be of use in an occasional patient.

Methotrexate

Methotrexate is presently the SAARD most often prescribed by rheumatologists. It has been extensively studied and its side effects well characterized. It is generally given as a low-dose weekly pulse, initially at about 7.5 mg/wk. In contrast to many SAARDs, many patients report clinical improvement within several weeks after starting the drug and response plateaus over about 12 weeks. For patients not responding to the initial dose, incremental doses usually will result in improvement.

Most of the side effects of methotrexate are dose dependent and include:

- Mucositis
- Nausea and vomiting
- Diarrhea.

Patients with low folate levels may be more susceptible to methotrexate toxicity. The addition of folic acid and low-dose folinic acid appear to circumvent some of the toxicity without reducing efficacy. Some patients report a troubling post-dose malaise that can last several days, making therapy with this compound difficult. A rare patient will develop acute pulmonary symptoms after starting methotrexate with fever, hypoxia, and infiltrates observed on chest radiographs. The risk of hepatic dysfunction in association with methotrexate is rare, but most rheumatologists do monitor transaminases during therapy. Finally, methotrexate is handled by the kidney, and major dose adjustments may be necessary in patients with renal dysfunction.

Anticytokines

The inflammatory cytokine TNF-α has been shown to play an important role in the pathogenesis of RA. Recently, two compounds have become available which interfere with TNF.

The first agent, a chimeric monoclonal antibody, infliximab, directed against TNF-α (but not against lympotoxin, TNF-β), neutralizes TNF-α and rapidly produces improvement in the signs and symptoms of RA and slows radiographic progression of the disease. It is administered as three loading doses and then is generally given every other month. It has been approved for treatment of RA patients who are also on methotrexate. Human anti-chimera antibodies do develop in some patients treated with infliximab, but they occur less often in patients treated with concomitant methotrexate. In most patients, infliximab is well tolerated. Mild, but not serious infections, are seen more often in patients treated with infliximab as is the development of certain autoantibodies.

Etanercept is another new agent for the treatment of RA. This protein is a soluble receptor for TNF-α and TNF-β. It is administered subcutaneously twice weekly. Etanercept is effective and frequently used alone or in conjunction with methotrexate in patients who have active disease despite methotrexate alone. Treatment with etanercept also appears to slow radiographic progression of RA. Most tolerate this compound well, although an occasional patient may develop a local reaction. Patients who develop infections while on etanercept should discontinue its use until the infection clears.

■ Hydroxychloroquine

Hydroxychloroquine is the most commonly used antimalarial drug to treat RA and is frequently used to treat patients with mild disease. The initial dose is 200 mg bid, although higher doses are occasionally used. Joint pain and swelling and morning stiffness are improved with this compound, but it is unclear if it alters radiographic disease progression. The antirheumatic mechanism of these compounds is not known, but they may elevate intracellular pH and perhaps interfere with antigen presentation.

The drug is generally well tolerated, but the onset of action may be delayed for several months after the drug is initiated. Retinal toxicity is a rare complication, usually seen when doses of greater than 6.5 mg/kg/d are used, but generally readily recognized with regular fundoscopic examinations.

■ Sulfasalazine

Sulfasalazine is another compound which has been found to be effective in RA. Interestingly, in contrast to many agents which were coincidentally found to be effective in RA, sulfasalazine was actually designed to treat RA. It is a combination of both a salicylate and a sulfa drug. The moiety responsible for sulfasalazine action is not known; indeed, the overall mechanism of action is unclear.

Therapy is generally initiated with an incremental dosing scheme going up to about 2000 mg/d. In direct comparisons with penicillamine, sulfasalazine was equally effective, but response was quicker. Similarly, when compared to injectable gold, sulfasalazine was found to be equally effective. Generally, patients do not respond for 2 to 3 months after initiating therapy.

Sulfasalazine is also generally well tolerated, particularly the enteric-coated form. In addition to GI toxicity (nausea and anorexia), some patients develop malaise and fever. Occasionally, a patient will develop a rash or leukopenia. These side effects are usually seen early in the course of therapy. Sulfasalazine also interferes with folate metabolism and may lead to a megaloblastic anemia.

■ Gold Salts

Gold salts, either injectable or the oral form, auranofin, have largely been supplanted by other agents, particularly methotrexate. Nonetheless, these compounds are effective and may be of use for the treatment of an occasional patient. *In vitro* studies have demonstrated that gold compounds have effects on B cells, antigen presentation, and lymphocyte mitogenic response, among others. Which, if any, of these effects are important *in vivo* is not known. Approximately two thirds of patients treated with injectable gold will respond. Typically, patients will note:

- Decreased morning stiffness
- Decreased painful and swollen joints
- Declined laboratory measures of disease activity.

14

Moreover, injectable gold slows the radiographic progression of the disease.

Common gold toxicities include:
- Pruritic rashes
- Cytopenias
- Proteinuria.

Most physicians will monitor a urinanalysis and blood count carefully during therapy. The renal lesion due to gold is similar to that seen in idiopathic membranous nephritis.

Injectable gold is often given as an initial test dose of about 10 to 25 mg followed by a loading dose of 50 mg/wk, until 1000 mg have been given. As with many other slow-acting agents, response to injectable gold may require months of therapy. Patients who respond can be maintained on every-other-week, or even less frequent, injections.

Oral gold or auranofin is better tolerated than injectable gold, but may be less effective. Studies evaluating patients who had been maintained on injectable gold who were then switched to oral gold frequently experienced a flare of their arthritis. In addition, some patients started on auranofin may note a dose-related diarrhea which can surmounted by a slow-dose increment and a high-fiber diet.

■ Penicillamine

Penicillamine is a sulfhydryl analog of cysteine and, because of the sulfhydryl moiety, is capable of binding divalent cations which may modulate protease and oxidant production and potentially limit tissue damage. Therapy with penicillamine is effective in RA and results in improvement of fatigue, joint signs and symptoms, and laboratory measures of disease activity. Overall, it is comparable to compounds such as azathioprine and gold.

The starting dose of penicillamine is typically 250 mg/d and is slowly incremented to the range of 750 to 1000 mg. The drug should not be given with food, since it interferes with absorption. A therapeutic response may not be seen for 6 months.

Toxicity and the availability of other more readily tolerated agents has, to a large extent, relegated the use of penicillamine in RA to the history books. Patients treated with penicillamine often note dysgeusia, which usually resolves with continued therapy. Cytopenias, proteinuria, and usually pruritus rashes are the most common side effects. Perhaps even more troublesome is the appearance of autoimmune disorders during penicillamine therapy, including:

- Myasthenia gravis
- Myositis
- Lupus.

■ Other Therapies and Combinations

A number of other agents has been used to treat patients with RA. Some of the more commonly employed include azathioprine, cyclosporin A, and thalidomide (which requires special Food and Drug Administration approval). Each of these has been found to be effective therapies, but do require special monitoring. Similarly, alkylating agents such as cyclophosphamide and chlorambucil are quite effective, but their toxicities, including myelodysplasia and the development of certain malignancies, have relegated these agents for use in patients with aggressive disease that has not responded to other available therapies.

Over the last several years, trials (frequently open-labeled) of combination SAARDs have been completed. Since the mechanisms of action of these compounds are largely not known, their choice in combinations have largely been empiric. Concerns have been raised about the additional costs and potential toxicities of the combinations. Despite this, two

14

combinations show some promise. The addition of cyclosporin A to patients on methotrexate does improve the response. In selected patients, methotrexate with hydroxychloroquine and sulfasalazine may be more effective than the same dose of methotrexate alone. Further studies are needed to fully assess the benefit of these combinations.

■ Experimental Therapies

There has been an explosion of new therapeutic agents for the treatment of RA. Many of the initial agents have targeted lymphocytes with monoclonal antibodies directed against cell-surface markers. For the most part, these therapies have been ineffective. These results have led to a reexamination of the fundamental processes involved in the tissue injury and clinical manifestations of the disease.

Protease inhibitors should directly block the enzymatic resorption of cartilage and subjacent bone, but their critical role in normal tissue turnover and wound healing may limit their application. Protease production and the regulation of the balance between cartilage production and degradation is in part mediated by a number of inflammatory cytokines. Perhaps most prominent, TNF-α upregulates a number of proteolytic enzymes and induces production of other cytokines such as IL-1 and IL-6. As noted above, interference with the effects of TNF-α has been shown to be effective in the treatment of RA. Other compounds are being developed which should interfere with either its (TNF) effect or release, and should add to our therapies for RA.

Other agents, including administration of IL-4 or IL-10 as regulatory cytokines or interference with action of inducible ICAM-1 or production of IL-1, are among other therapies presently being evaluated for treatment of RA.

Surgical Therapy

Articular surgical procedures for patients with RA are often reserved for those patients whose disease is not controlled with medical regimens, or in which joint damage interferes with function or causes unremitting pain. In selected patients, synovectomy is helpful. An example might be a patient with unremitting elbow disease who has ulnar nerve impingement, recognizing that the disease is likely to recur if medical management cannot control the disease.

Total joint arthroplasty has revolutionized care of patients with certain failed joints. In most, pain is the leading indicator for surgical intervention. Preoperatively, it is important to identify and correct, if possible, potential risk factors. Skin lesions near the joint should be healed and other potential sites for bacterial seeding of the prosthesis (eg, prostatism [in males], urinary tract and sinus infections) should be evaluated and treated. Hip and knee prosthesis are the best studied. Most can expect the prosthesis to last for about 15 years. Shoulder arthroplasty is also useful for relieving pain. In many rheumatoid patients, there is resorption of the rotator cuff, which limits range of motion, even with the prosthetic device. Of course, axial loading of the arm has to be limited after the device is in place.

Hand surgery is usually employed to improve lost function. There is no reason to operate on a functional, pain-free hand, despite the extent of cosmetic deformities. Other procedures, such as ankle fusions and metatarsal transection, are occasionally useful and should be planned in conjunction with other providers.

SUGGESTED READING

American College of Rheumatology Ad Hoc Committee on Clinical Guidelines. Guidelines for monitoring drug therapy in rheumatoid arthritis. *Arthritis Rheum.* 1996;39:723-731.

American College of Rheumatology Ad Hoc Committee on Clinical Guidelines. Guidelines for the management of rheumatoid arthritis. *Arthritis Rheum.* 1996;39:713-722.

Arnett FC, Edworthy SM, Bloch DA, et al. The American Rheumatism Association 1987 revised criteria for the classification of rheumatoid arthritis. *Arthritis Rheum.* 1988;31:315-324.

Bensen WG, Agrawal N, Zhao S, et al. Upper gastrointestinal tolerability of celecoxib: a Cox-2 specific inhibitor, compared to naproxen and placebo. *Arthritis Rheum.* 1999;42:S142.

Bensen WG, Fiechtner JJ, McMillen JI, et al. Treatment of osteoarthritis with celecoxib, a cyclooxygenase-2 inhibitor. A randomized control trial. *Mayo Clin Proc.* 1999;74:1095-1105.

Blackburn WD Jr. Validity of acute phase proteins as markers of disease activity. *J Rheumatol.* 1994;21(suppl):9-13.

Harris ED Jr. Rheumatoid arthritis: the clinical spectrum. In: Kelley WN, Harris ED Jr, Rubby S, eds. *Textbook of Rheumatology.* Vol 1. 4th ed. Philadelphia, Pa: WB Saunders Company; 1981:932.

Kremer JM, Alarcón G, Lightfoot RW Jr, et al. Methotrexate for rheumatoid arthritis. Suggested guidelines for monitoring liver toxicity. American College of Rheumatology. *Arthritis Rheum.* 1994; 37:316-328.

O'Sullivan JB, Cathcart RD. The prevalence of rheumatoid arthritis. Follow-up evaluation of the effect of criteria on rates in Sudbury, Massachusetts. *Ann Intern Med.* 1972;76:573-576.

Singh G, Ramey D, Triadafilopoulos G. Early experience with selective Cox-2 inhibitors, safety profile in over 340,000 patient years of use. *Arthritis Rheum.* 1999;42:S296.

Simon LS, Weaver AL, Graham DY, et al. Anti-inflammatory and upper gastrointestinal effects of celecoxib in rheumatoid arthritis. A randomized controlled trial. *JAMA.* 1999;283:1921-1928.

15 Scleroderma

Scleroderma, or "hard skin," is an inflammatory disorder which leads to fibrosis of involved skin and viscera. Also referred to as systemic sclerosis, based on clinical and antibody profiles, it is further segregated into either a diffuse or limited form.

Pathogenesis

The cause of and factors leading to the development of the clinical syndrome called scleroderma are not known, but any theory regarding the pathogenesis must explain the:

- Increased deposition of collagen
- Vascular changes
- Presence of certain autoantibodies.

Vascular abnormalities, as evidenced by basement membrane thickening and endothelial damage, are visible early in the course of the disease. Fibroblasts produce excess collagen, but these changes appear to be in response to exogenous signals.

Autoantibodies in certain subsets of antinuclear antibodies are present in nearly all patients with scleroderma. Of interest, the presence of anti-centromere antibodies has been associated with the presence of human leukocyte antigen (HLA)-DQB1*0501, *0301, and *0402, whereas anti-topoisomerase I antibodies have been linked to HLA-DQB1*0301. Whether these antibodies play a role in initiating or perpetuating the disease is unclear.

A number of reports have been published linking scleroderma to certain environmental exposures.

Fortunately, careful epidemiological studies have laid many of these issues to rest. This is certainly the case regarding silicone breast implants, where abundant evidence clearly indicates no association between implants and the development of scleroderma. Silica has been held as an example of environmentally induced scleroderma. However, this conclusion has been based on anecdotal reports. More recent comparison studies demonstrate no association between systemic sclerosis and silica exposure.

A "scleroderma-like" syndrome has been described in patients in Spain who had ingested an adulterated cooking oil; however, this syndrome is distinct from scleroderma. Initial reports have also linked what has been termed eosinophilic myalgia syndrome with exposure to l-tryptophan, but the validity of this conclusion remains questionable.

Occurrence

Scleroderma is a relatively rare disorder. Prevalence figures have ranged from about 29 to 113 per 100,000. Hennekens and colleagues reported that the prevalence of self-reported scleroderma was 1 of 1225 women or a prevalence of 82 per 100,000. Maricq and colleagues evaluated nearly 7000 individuals in South Carolina and estimated that scleroderma spectrum disorders occurred in 67 to 265 per 100,000 population.

Clinical Features

The most characteristic clinical features of scleroderma are the skin changes, such as:

- Initially, the skin is edematous with diffuse puffiness and patients note stiffness (Figure 15.1).

FIGURE 15.1 — PUFFY SKIN OF SCLERODERMA

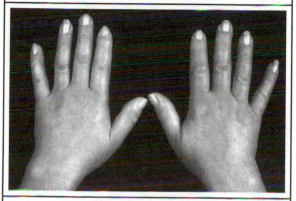

Diffuse puffiness of the hands, which may be seen early in patients with scleroderma. This may give way in a matter of weeks to the taut skin more diagnostic of scleroderma.

Courtesy of the Arthritis Foundation.

- Over a variable period of time, frequently months, the puffiness is replaced by skin thickening (Figure 15.2).
- In those individuals with limited scleroderma, skin changes are usually limited to the fingers, hands, and face.
- These changes may be also associated with subcutaneous calcifications, which may be palpable or visualized radiographically.
- Patients with diffuse disease will have skin changes more proximally on the arms, as well as the legs and trunk.
- Sweat glands and hair follicles are lost from the involved skin and the skin may take on a sometimes dramatic "salt and pepper" hyperpigmentation.

15

FIGURE 15.2 — TIGHT, THICKENING SKIN OF SCLERODERMA

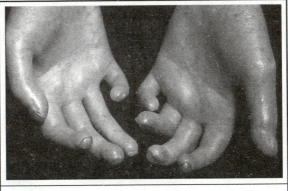

Courtesy of the Arthritis Foundation.

At this phase, motion may also be restricted. Fine movements of the fingers may be impaired. Those with involvement around the mouth may have problems with eating and oral hygiene. Patients with diffuse disease often note progression of the skin changes for a year or two. Skin over bony prominences is stretched and contractures may develop. Skin ulcers may develop over the tufts of the distal phalanges or over other bony prominences that are difficult to heal (Figure 15.3). Over time, skin may soften and, apart from appendage loss, pigmentation, and development of telangiectasia (Figure 15.4), may be difficult to recognize as sclerodermatous skin.

Although the skin changes are most typical and necessary for diagnosis, other features of scleroderma are often associated with morbidity or mortality. Raynaud's phenomenon, or abnormal vasospasm to cold or stress, involves a triphasic response of pallor, cyanosis, and erythema with rewarming. Nearly all patients with scleroderma will experience Raynaud's. It can range from being an annoyance to severe enough to cause digital necrosis.

FIGURE 15.3 — SKIN ULCERS FORMING OVER TUFTS OF DISTAL PHALANGES IN SCLERODERMA

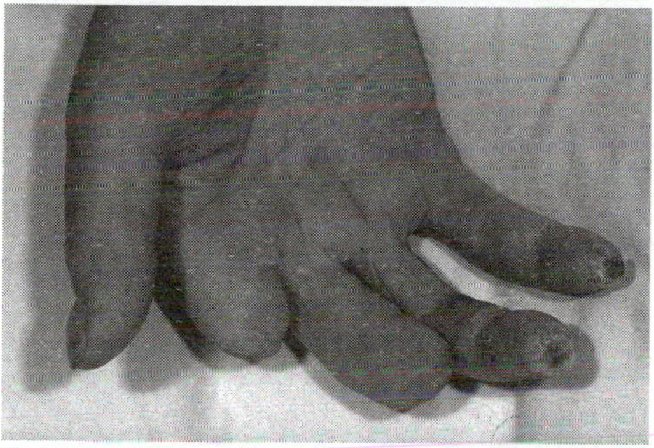

Courtesy of Gower Medical Publishing Ltd.

Pulmonary involvement is presently the most common cause of morbidity in patients with scleroderma. About two thirds of patients will have lung involvement that may be manifest as a nonproductive cough and/or dyspnea. Examination of the chest reveals dry rales, and chest radiographs will demonstrate evidence of interstitial fibrosis. Abnormalities in a pulmonary function test include restrictive changes and a reduced diffusing capacity. Varying degrees of pulmonary hypertension may be apparent. An occasional patient will develop pulmonary hypertension in the absence of significant interstitial fibrosis. This is rapidly progressive with dyspnea and right-sided heart failure. Early and more rapidly progressive pulmonary disease is seen more often in patients with diffuse disease than in those with localized scleroderma.

The gastrointestinal (GI) tract may be involved anywhere from the mouth to the rectum. As noted above, skin involvement around the mouth may limit its opening. However, esophageal dysfunction is the

201

FIGURE 15.4 — TELANGIECTASIA OF SCLERODERMA

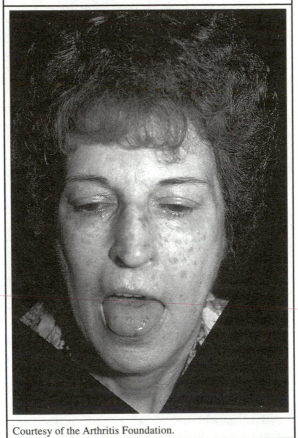

Courtesy of the Arthritis Foundation.

most common form of GI involvement and occurs in either the limited or diffuse form of the disease. Insufficiency of the gastroesophageal sphincter leads to reflux, symptoms of heartburn, and, in some, esophageal stricture. In addition, sclerodermatous involvement of the lower esophagus leads to poor propulsion and dysphagia, initially for solids. Symptomatic small-bowel involvement occurs in the minority of patients. Fibrosis of the small bowel leads to hypomotility, cramping and bloating. This may be further exacerbated by overgrowth with intestinal bacteria, the development of malabsorption, and diarrhea. Involvement of the colon is more common than of the small bowel. Wide-mouth-saccular diverticuli, representing colonic involvement, are often simply a radiographic curiosity. However, they can be associated with constipation, impaction and, rarely, perforation.

Renal involvement, previously a common cause of mortality in scleroderma, is seen almost exclusively in patients with diffuse disease. Patients present with severe hypertension, which may develop abruptly in association with renal dysfunction. Visualization of renal vessels has disclosed marked constriction of interlobular arteries and diminished glomerular perfusion, accounting for the high renin states. Untreated, progressive azotemia ensues.

Musculoskeletal complaints are common in patients with scleroderma, but frank synovitis is unusual. Joint pain and stiffness can often be attributed to skin thickening or involvement of tendons. Friction rubs can be heard and even occasionally palpated.

Coronary vessels undergo vasospasm in scleroderma patients in response to similar stimuli that induce digital artery vasospasm and may be associated with left ventricular dysfunction. Pericardial effusions are frequently detectable with echocardiograms but rarely are large enough to impair ventricular filling. More frequent cardiac changes are secondary to lung disease or hypertension.

Laboratory Tests and Radiographs

As with many rheumatic diseases, there are few tests specific for scleroderma. If adequate substrates are used, antinuclear antibodies (ANAs) are found in over 90% of patients. Specific ANAs are related to the scleroderma clinical presentation. Scl-70 antibodies (anti-topoisomerase I) are present in sera of about one third of individuals with diffuse scleroderma, but in only about 10% of those with limited disease. In contrast, anticentromere antibodies are found in about half of those with limited disease and rarely in those with diffuse scleroderma. A similar association has been found between anti-Th and limited scleroderma and anti-RNA polymerase III and diffuse disease. The role, if any, of these antibodies in the disease process remains unclear.

Other laboratory tests and radiographs are used to determine the extent or progression of the disease. Diffusing capacity may be the first of the pulmonary function tests affected by scleroderma. Chest radiographs may be normal early or show progressive interstitial fibrosis. Esophageal manometry or barium swallowing studies may detect GI involvement. Routine chemistries are useful for detecting and following renal function abnormalities. Other tests, such as echocardiograms, may be of some utility in those with pulmonary hypertension or pericardial disease.

Diagnosis

The diagnosis of scleroderma is dependent upon finding skin changes on physical examination. Criteria have been developed by the American College of Rheumatology (Table 15.1). In most individuals who have established skin changes, the diagnosis is not a challenge. In earlier disease, the diffuse puffiness can be confused with the diffuse swelling sometimes seen in the seronegative spondyloarthropathies (SNSAs). The thickened skin caused by years of manual labor may be difficult to differentiate from limited scleroderma.

TABLE 15.1 — AMERICAN RHEUMATISM ASSOCIATION SCLERODERMA CRITERIA COOPERATIVE STUDY: PRELIMINARY CLINICAL CRITERIA FOR SYSTEMIC SCLEROSIS*

- Proximal scleroderma is the single major criterion; sensitivity was 91% and specificity was over 99%.
- Sclerodactyly (digital pitting scars of fingertips or loss of substance of the distal finger pad) and bibasilar pulmonary fibrosis contributed further as minor criteria in the absence of proximal scleroderma
- One major or two or more minor criteria were found in 97% of definite systemic sclerosis patients, but only in 2% of the comparison patients with systemic lupus erythematosus, polymyositis/dermatomyositis, or Raynaud's phenomenon

* Excludes localized scleroderma and pseudosclerodermatous disorders.

Subcommittee for scleroderma criteria of the American Rheumatism Association Diagnostic and Therapeutic Criteria Committee. *Arthritis Rheum.* 1980;23:581-590.

Management

Over the years, numerous drugs have been tried as primary treatment for scleroderma. Often, reports of success have come from uncontrolled, unblinded anecdotes, which are later refuted by carefully controlled, blinded studies. Perhaps the most recent example is penicillamine. Long held out as a potential therapy for scleroderma, recent blinded studies have not shown efficacy, and it does have significant toxicity. Nonetheless, there are many interventions that can provide, at the least, symptomatic relief. Range of motion exercises and careful attention to skin ulcers limits contractures and complications of digital ulcers.

15

Treatment of GI complications is often beneficial. Decreases in the oral aperture may be overcome by exercise and complications limited by good oral hygiene. Problems with dysphagia and the associated reflux can be treated with H_2-blockers or proton-pump inhibitors with dramatic relief. Malabsorption due to small-bowel overgrowth can be treated with antibiotics. Painful Raynaud's phenomenon can be treated by a number of means. The simplest is warm clothing and gloves in cold weather. A number of other agents have had some success, including topical nitrates and vasodilators. Calcium channel blockers, particularly those that have a peripheral vasodilatory effect, are perhaps the most useful for treating Raynaud's.

Pulmonary disease is particularly difficult to treat. Prudent recommendations include exercise and discontinuation of cigarette smoking. Prostacyclin infusions may be helpful in decreasing pulmonary arterial pressures, but this is expensive, cumbersome, and reverses once the infusion is stopped.

Previously associated with significant mortality, scleroderma renal crisis is now usually readily treated with angiotensin-converting enzyme inhibitors. In most patients, blood pressure can be controlled with these agents and often azotemia reversed. Nonetheless, an occasional patient may develop renal failure due to scleroderma, and dialysis may become necessary. Access may be difficult depending upon the extent of skin involvement.

Arthritis may well be controlled with nonsteroidal anti-inflammatory drugs or with low-dose corticosteroids. Steroids are sometimes employed in patients with aggressive skin disease or with active pulmonary scleroderma, but their use is at best empiric.

SUGGESTED READING

Hennekens CH, Lee IM, Cook NR, et al. Self-reported breast implants and connective-tissue diseases in female health professionals. A retrospective cohort. *JAMA*. 1996;275:616-621.

LeRoy EC, Black C, Fleischmajer R, et al. Scleroderma (systemic sclerosis): classification, subsets and pathogenesis. *J Rheumatol*. 1988;15:202-205.

Maricq HR, Weinrich MC, Keil JE, et al. Prevalence of scleroderma spectrum disorders in the general population of South Carolina. *Arthritis Rheum*. 1989;32:998-1006.

Reimer G, Steen VD, Penning CA, Medsger TA Jr, Tan EM. Correlates between autoantibodies to nucleolar antigens and clinical features in patients with systemic sclerosis (scleroderma). *Arthritis Rheum*. 1988;31:525-532.

Steen VD, Blari S, Medsger TA Jr. The toxicity of D-penicillamine in systemic sclerosis. *Ann Intern Med*. 1986;104:699-705.

Steen VD, Costantino JP, Shapiro AP, Medsger TA Jr. Outcome of renal crisis in systemic sclerosis: relation to availability to angiotensin-converting enzyme (ACE) inhibitors. *Ann Intern Med*. 1990;113:352-357.

Subcommittee for Scleroderma Criteria of the American Rheumatism Association Diagnostic and Therapeutic Criteria Committee. Preliminary criteria for the classification of systemic sclerosis (scleroderma). *Arthritis Rheum*. 1980;23:581-590.

Winterbauer R. Multiple telangiectasia, Raynaud's phenomenon, sclerodactyly, and subcutaneous calcinosis: a syndrome mimicking hereditary telangiectasia. *Bull Johns Hopkins Hosp*. 1964;114: 361-383.

15

16   Septic Arthritis

Septic arthritis is usually the most worrisome consideration when patients present with a warm, swollen joint. Bacterial invasion of a joint can rapidly lead to irreversible cartilage resorption and, in some cases, to sepsis and death. Access to the joint by the infecting organism most often occurs via hematogenous spread, but may penetrate the joint during the course of a contiguous osteomyelitis or be introduced into the joint by trauma or joint manipulation.

The clinical presentation is determined by both the organism involved and specific host factors. One host factor in particular, namely a preexisting arthritis, may cause confusion and delay in diagnosis. Table 16.1 contains a listing of the more common organisms associated with septic arthritis, the presently recommended antibiotic choices, and the populations at risk. Final antibiotic selection should take into consideration local information regarding drug sensitivity.

In general, optimal treatment of septic arthritis includes:

- Collection of appropriate cultures prior to initiating antibiotics
- Early and appropriate antibiotic therapy
- Adequate joint drainage.

In addition to culture of joint fluids, blood cultures and cultures of other sites may be necessary to affect a bacteriological diagnosis. Antibiotic therapy is often initiated empirically and guided by subsequent culture results. Most often, joint drainage can be accomplished with simple and repeated needle aspiration. When the hip is involved, open drainage may

TABLE 16.1 — CAUSES, TREATMENT AND AFFECTED POPULATIONS OF SEPTIC ARTHRITIS

Population Affected	Etiologies	Suggested Regimens	
		Primary	Alternative
Infant < 3 months	*Staphylococcus aureus*, Enterobacteriaceae, group B streptococci	PRSP + P Ceph 3	PRSP + APAG (If MRSA prevalent, vanco in place of PRSP)
Children (3 months to 6 years)	*S aureus* (35%), *Haemophilus influenzae* (15%), streptococci (10%), Enterobacteriaceae (6%)	PRSP + P Ceph 3	Vanco for PRSP
Adult	*S aureus* (40%), group A streptococci (27%), Enterobacteriaceae (27%)	[(PRSP or P Ceph 1) + (APAG or CIP)] or TC/CL or PIP/TZ or AM/SB	Vanco for PRSP, CIP + RIF
Adult, rheumatoid	*S aureus* (74%), streptococci (16%), Enterobacteriaceae (8%)	PRSP or P Ceph 1	Vanco or CIP + RIF or TC/CL or PIP/TZ or AM/SB

| Prosthetic joint, post-operative, post intra-articular injection | S epidermidis (40%), S aureus (20%), Enterobacteriaceae, Pseudomonas species | Vanco + CIP (or aztreonam or APAG) | CIP 750 mg po bid + RIF 900 mg po qd or oflox 200 mg po tid + RIF 900 mg po qd |

Abbreviations: PRSP, penicillinase-resistant synthetic penicillin; P Ceph 3, third-generation parenteral cephalosporin; APAG, antipseudomonal aminoglycosidic antibiotic; MRSA, methicillin-resistant *Staphylococcus aureus*; P Ceph 1, first-generation parenteral cephalosporin; vanco, vancomycin; CIP, ciprofloxacin; RIF, rifampin; TC/CL, ticarcillin/clavulanate (Timentin); PIP/TZ, piperacillin/tazobactam; AM/SB, ampicillin/sulbactam (Unasyn); oflox, ofloxacin.

Adapted from: Sanford JP, et al. *The Sanford Guide to Antimicrobial Therapy, 1998.* 1998:21-22.

16

be necessary. In other joints when needle aspiration and antibiotic therapy does not lead to clinical improvement, arthroscopic or other drainage procedures may be needed.

Many other organisms have been occasionally implicated, underscoring the importance of adequate collection of cultures. The discussion of the more common or characteristic organisms associated with joint infections follows below.

Septic Arthritis in Childhood

Organisms responsible for septic arthritis in children vary considerably depending upon the age of the child. It is also more often linked to osteomyelitis, because of the open epiphyses. In newborns, it is most likely to be due to either *Staphylococcus aureus*, *group B streptococci* or, less often, gram-negative organisms. The hips, knees and ankles are most often involved.

Septic arthritis in children between 6 months and 24 months also predominantly involves the large joints of the legs and has historically been due to *Haemophilus influenzae* and *Kingella kingae*. Immunization has reduced *H influenzae* infections, but they still represent an important consideration. Organisms responsible for septic arthritis in older children more closely resemble those seen in adults. Gonococcal arthritis is a consideration in the older, sexually active child.

Septic Arthritis in Adults

The most common cause of septic arthritis is *Neisseria gonorrhoeae* and it is a manifestation of disseminated gonococcal infection (DGI). Patients are usually younger and sexually active. Women develop DGI more often than men, which may be related to the fact that they more often have chronic subclinical urethritis. Additionally, dissemination seems to oc-
212

cur more often during menstruation, a time when there is ready access to the blood stream.

Many patients may not report symptoms of urethritis, but if present, is a clue to the source of dissemination. The arthritis is initially migratory, frequently involving several joints at once, and usually associated with an impressive tenosynovitis. Fever, although it may be low-grade, is generally present. After several days, the arthritis may localize to one or more joints, such as the knee, hip or wrist, and will become increasingly symptomatic. In about half of patients with DGI, a pustular skin rash will be present (Figure 16.1) which, although characteristic, may be seen with other organisms, particularly *N meningitidis*.

FIGURE 16.1 — PUSTULAR SKIN RASH OF DISSEMINATED GONOCOCCAL INFECTION

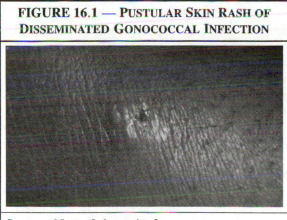

Courtesy of Syntex Laboratories, Inc.

16

Synovial fluid will usually have an elevated white blood cell count, but organisms are difficult to retrieve in culture (less than half the time) and are even less often seen on Gram stain. Cultures obtained from the oral, urethral or rectal mucosa are more likely to aid in the establishment of the diagnosis. Recently, polymerase chain reaction-based assays have become available that should enhance diagnostic capabilities.

Treatment is usually started empirically, based on the clinical setting and assisted by Gram stain results. Initiation of antibiotic therapy early in the course will generally lead to a rapid and complete resolution of symptoms. Delay in therapy may be associated with irreversible cartilage damage.

In most situations, septic arthritis due to *S aureus* is a monoarthritis and the knee is the most commonly affected joint. Risk factors include:

- Older age
- Another form of arthritis
- A prosthetic joint
- Intravenous drug use
- Therapy with corticosteroids
- Other immunosuppressive conditions.

Early detection, aggressive drainage, and appropriate antibiotics for *S aureus* septic arthritis is particularly important if a good outcome is to ensue, as infection with this virulent organism rapidly leads to joint destruction. The emergence of methicillin-resistant *S aureus* has led to the use of vancomycin as the drug of choice when this organism is suspected. Since few other alternatives are available, careful consideration should be given regarding when, at what dose, and how long this antibiotic is used.

S epidermidis is a common, not-to-be-overlooked cause of prosthetic joint infections or joint infection in the elderly. Infection of the prosthetic joint by this organism is generally seen early after the prosthesis is placed and, in the appropriate clinical setting, should not be considered a laboratory contaminant. Appropriate antibiotic therapy may lead to clearing of the infection, but prosthesis loss is common.

Group B and group G streptococcal joint infections occur in adults, particularly those with other complicating medical illnesses, including diabetes mellitus, rheumatoid arthritis and alcoholism. These

214

organisms may present as an isolated monoarthritis, but also have been causes of polyarthritis.

Streptococcal pneumoniae may cause septic arthritis, generally in association with other infections such as pneumonia or meningitis. Joint seeding is thought to occur hematogenously. In the alcoholic or the patient with hypogammaglobulinemia, joint sepsis may be polyarticular.

Depending upon the population studied, 10% or more of the cases of septic arthritis are due to gram-negative bacilli. The elderly and those with rheumatoid arthritis are particularly susceptible. Abdominal or genitourinary sources are usually implicated, and organisms such as *Escherichia coli* and *Proteus mirabilis* are the more common gram-negative isolates. Infection of prosthetic joints due to gram-negative organisms generally leads to removal of the hardware. Intravenous drug use is a risk factor for gram-negative septic arthritis. In this group of patients, coliforms are again often the causative organisms. Additionally, the joints infected may include the sternoclavicular or sacroiliac joints: joints uncommonly involved in other clinical settings. *Pasteurella multocida* is a small gram-negative coccobacillus found on the oral mucosa of many domestic animals. This usually penicillin-sensitive organism is a consideration when septic arthritis occurs after a cat or dog bite or scratch.

SUGGESTED READING

16

Blackburn WD Jr, Dunn TL, Alarcón GS. Infection versus disease activity in rheumatoid arthritis: eight years' experience. *South Med J.* 1986;79:1238-1241.

Goldenberg DL. Bacterial arthritis. *Curr Opin Rheumatol.* 1995;7: 310-314.

O'Brien JP, Goldenberg DL, Rice PA. Disseminated gonococcal infections: a prospective analysis of 49 patients and a review of pathophysiology and immune mechanisms. *Medicine*. 1983;62: 395-406.

Rosenthal J, Bole GG, Robinson WD. Acute nongonococcal infectious arthritis. Evaluation of risk factors, therapy, and outcome. *Arthritis Rheum*. 1980;23:889-897.

Sanford JP, Moellering RC Jr, Gilbert DN. *The Sanford Guide to Antimicrobial Therapy, 1998*. Vienna, Va: Antimicrobial Therapy, Inc; 1998.

17 Soft Tissue Rheumatism

Pain derived from specific soft tissue structures is perhaps the most common reason for patients to seek care for musculoskeletal problems. Essentially every person will experience soft-tissue rheumatism. In most situations, the pain is related to or exacerbated by use or trauma and, in isolation, is rarely indicative of a systemic rheumatic disorder. In the same light, treatment of soft-tissue rheumatism, in contrast to many systemic rheumatic diseases, can be gratifying, often with rapid and long-lasting relief. There are many soft-tissue structures which have been associated with painful syndromes. The most common are discussed here.

Hand

de Quervain's tenosynovitis is inflammation of the abductor pollicis longus and extensor pollicis brevis at their insertion sites at the base of the thumb (Figure 17.1). Patients often give a history of performing tasks where there is frequent movement of the thumb in a radial direction. Pressure over the tendon and the Finkelstein test, grasping the thumb with the fingers in the palm of the hand and moving the hand ulnarly, elicits pain. At times, it may be difficult differentiating pain from this tendon from pain due to osteoarthritis of the carpometacarpal joint. Treatment involves rest of the tendon and alteration of the task which causes pain. Injection of steroids along the tendon sheath is often useful.

Flexor or extensor tenosynovitis is occasionally responsible for hand pain unrelated to another disor-

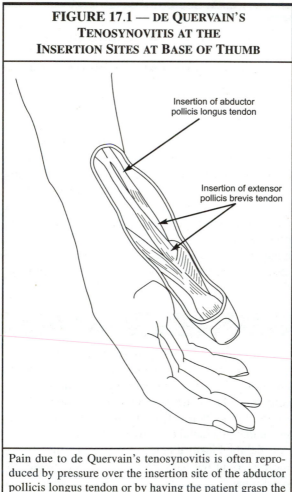

Insertion of abductor
pollicis longus tendon

Insertion of extensor
pollicis brevis tendon

Pain due to de Quervain's tenosynovitis is often reproduced by pressure over the insertion site of the abductor pollicis longus tendon or by having the patient grasp the thumb in the fingers of the same hand and moving the wrist in an ulnar direction.

der. Pain may be localized to the palm or dorsal aspect of the hand and worsened by resisted flexion or extension of the fingers (Figure 17.2). Rest is usually curative, but nonsteroidal anti-inflammatory drugs (NSAIDs) or injections can shorten the course. Ganglions are also encountered in association with the flexor or extensor tendons. These cystic structures may be painful or painless or simply a cosmetic concern. Ganglions can be aspirated and may resolve, but may require surgical removal.

Carpal tunnel syndrome is due to compression of the median nerve as it transverses the wrist. There, the median nerve passes deep to the palmaris longus tendon. The nerve provides sensory innervation to the palmar aspect of the thumb, index and middle fingers and motor innervation to most of the muscles of the thenar eminence. Patients often present with dysesthesia along the sensory distribution of the nerve, and frequently report pain to be worse at night. The Tinel's test, or tapping the wrist over the nerve, is considered positive if pain is elicited over the nerve's distribution. Similarly, the Phalen's maneuver reproduces symptoms with flexion of the wrist. The sensitivity and specificity of these tests are limited. Prolonged compression of the nerve may compromise motor function and thenar wasting may be evident.

Median nerve compression most often occurs in isolation, but may be due to inflammatory arthritis with compression due to infiltration of the synovium or associated with diabetes, amyloid or renal failure. In most, splinting in a neutral position, particularly at night, is ameliorative. Those who do not respond to splinting will often be afforded relief with steroid injections along the nerve. Development of muscle wasting is generally accepted as an indication for surgical intervention and decompression. Considerable forethought should be given prior to recommending surgery for patients with pain only, particularly if it

17

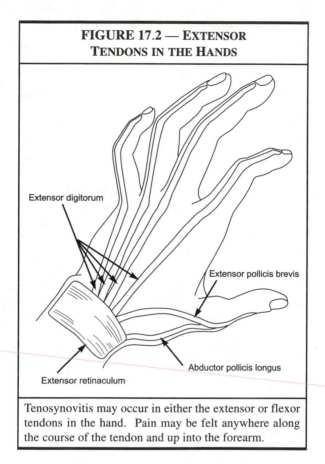

FIGURE 17.2 — EXTENSOR TENDONS IN THE HANDS

Extensor digitorum

Extensor pollicis brevis

Extensor retinaculum

Abductor pollicis longus

Tenosynovitis may occur in either the extensor or flexor tendons in the hand. Pain may be felt anywhere along the course of the tendon and up into the forearm.

does not follow the nerve's distribution or is associated with equivocal electrodiagnostic studies.

Ulnar nerve entrapment at the wrist is seen much less commonly than median nerve entrapment. It may present with sensory symptoms involving the fourth and fifth finger and/or weakness of apposition of the fourth and fifth fingers. The ulnar nerve also innervates the adductor pollicis, and injury to the nerve may be manifest by weakness in adduction of the thumb. The ulnar nerve may be damaged more proximally, particularly as it transverses the elbow in the condylar groove. Although ulnar nerve lesions may occur *de novo*, they are also seen in patients with disorders such as rheumatoid arthritis. Rest and padding the areas may be of use. Injections are sometimes used, particularly when there is synovium responsible for the nerve compression.

Elbow

Epicondylitis is diagnosed in patients who have elbow pain at the sites of origin of the wrist flexors or extensors (Figure 17.3). Lateral epicondylitis, often called tennis elbow, is characterized by tenderness localized to the lateral aspect of the elbow, which is usually worsened by resisted extension of the wrist. Although tennis players sometimes develop this, it is also seen in carpenters and individuals performing other activities in which there is forcible wrist extension. Medial epicondylitis or golfer's elbow is characterized by tenderness medially exacerbated by forcible wrist flexion. A number of remedies can be employed, including changing provocative activities, topical agents, NSAIDs, and local steroid injection. Injections give the most rapid relief. Acetaminophen can always be added as an analgesic and, as noted, has limited side effects.

Olecranon bursitis may be seen in association with rheumatoid arthritis, gout, and calcium pyrophosphate dihydrate (CPPD), after trauma, or due to infection. The bursa is swollen and may be warm and erythematous. Flexion of the elbow may cause pain, but supination and pronation usually do not. The bursa is easily aspirated and examination of the fluid is generally diagnostic. Bursal steroid injections are helpful for noninfectious conditions and appear to be more useful than NSAIDs. Acetaminophen can always be added as an analgesic.

17

FIGURE 17.3 — INSERTION SITES OF ARM FLEXORS

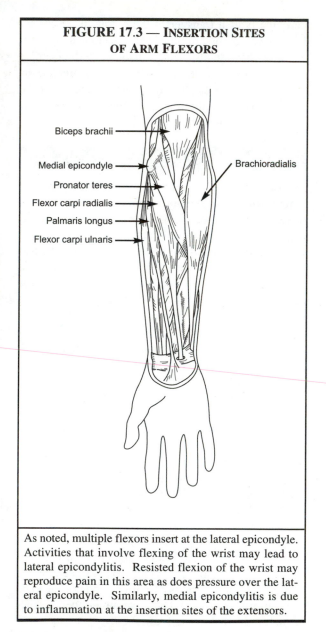

As noted, multiple flexors insert at the lateral epicondyle. Activities that involve flexing of the wrist may lead to lateral epicondylitis. Resisted flexion of the wrist may reproduce pain in this area as does pressure over the lateral epicondyle. Similarly, medial epicondylitis is due to inflammation at the insertion sites of the extensors.

A number of conditions may lead to pain which is perceived to be in the shoulder. Brachial neuritis, often idiopathic or linked to viral syndromes or trauma, can be recognized by the associated muscle weakness. Entrapment of the suprascapular nerve may lead to posterior shoulder pain and atrophy of this muscle over the scapula. Avascular necrosis of the humeral head may be linked to steroids, sickle cell disease, or trauma. Arthritis of the sternoclavicular or acromioclavicular joints may be confused with glenohumeral joint pain, but usually is easily differentiated on examination. Even poor posture is a cause of shoulder pain. Of course, visceral abnormalities, including Pancoast tumors and gall bladder, pulmonary, and cardiac disease, may lead to referred shoulder pain.

■ Common and Localized Shoulder Syndromes
Supraspinatus Tendinitis

Supraspinatus tendinitis usually presents as pain laterally in the shoulder (Figure 17.4). Frequently, symptoms cannot be distinguished from what some clinicians call subacromial bursitis.

The supraspinatus tendon receives its vascular supply from two areas:
- The fleshy belly of the muscle at its origin on the scapula
- Its attachment site on the humerus.

The tendon, as it courses under the acromion, has a tenuous vascular supply. When the shoulder is placed in abduction, the tendon may be impinged between the humerus and the acromium. On examination, there is tenderness localized over this point, which disappears under the acromion with abduction. With rupture, there may be a palpable deficit and weakness.

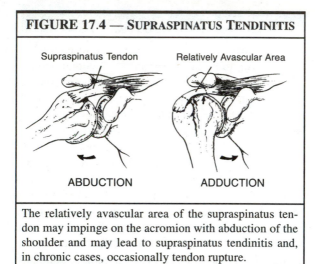

FIGURE 17.4 — SUPRASPINATUS TENDINITIS

Supraspinatus Tendon

Relatively Avascular Area

ABDUCTION

ADDUCTION

The relatively avascular area of the supraspinatus tendon may impinge on the acromion with abduction of the shoulder and may lead to supraspinatus tendinitis and, in chronic cases, occasionally tendon rupture.

Patients frequently report that pain is worse at night when they lie on the shoulder. Abduction of the shoulder to reach over the head or behind the back exacerbates symptoms. Younger patients often note prior activity where the hand is held over the head, such as swimming, pitching, carpentry, painting, or tennis. In older patients, similar activities exacerbate the symptoms and often those who push up to rise from a sitting position may develop similar symptoms. Patients may note that they can get their hand over their head by externally rotating the shoulder first, thereby rotating the supraspinatus tendon from under the acromion. Frequently, their symptoms may be chronic and rupture of the tendon limits their ability to abduct.

Calcific tendinitis tends to occur in middle-aged women who present with an acutely inflamed tendon, often with overlying erythema and, occasionally, fever. In these individuals, calcium crystals may be the etiologic factor.

Typically, plain radiographs of the shoulder are normal but, with chronic tendinitis, a subacromial traction spur may be apparent. Magnetic resonance imaging of the shoulder may reveal a tear.

A number of treatments have been recommended for supraspinatus tendinitis. Acutely, rest is usually prescribed. NSAIDs may be helpful, but response is often delayed. Steroid injections along the tendon sheath give immediate relief and are as successful as NSAIDs. Acetaminophen can always be added as an analgesic. Gradual rehabilitation probably limits the development of adhesive capsulitis. Pendulum exercises, advancing to full range of motion exercises with resistance, may be helpful. Younger patients with acute tears generally have them surgically repaired. Older patients with chronic tears, particularly if they are not painful, may be treated conservatively.

Bicipital Tendinitis

Bicipital tendinitis is due to irritation of the long head of the biceps as it rides over the humeral head (Figure 17.5). Pain is usually noted over the anterior shoulder and may actually radiate along the muscle to the forearm. In most patients, there are no clear inciting events. Activities that require resisted flexion of the elbow may exacerbate symptoms, as do abduction and internal rotation. Palpation of the bicipital tendon usually elicits pain. With the arm extended in front of the patient, resisted depression of the hand (Speed's test) elicits pain. With prolonged tendon irritation, it may become elongated and weakness of the biceps is noted. Rarely, there is rupture of the tendon. Acutely, this is painful and swollen. The biceps, tethered by its short head, is bunched over the mid-humerus, which is appropriately termed the "Popeye sign." Acute tendinitis is treated with rest and heat or cold. NSAIDs are often used, but injection along the tendon will give immediate relief and confirma-

17

FIGURE 17.5 — BICIPITAL TENDINITIS

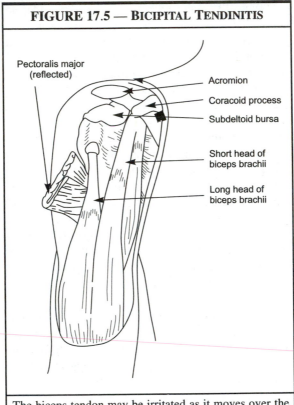

The biceps tendon may be irritated as it moves over the anterior humerus. Pain is localized to the tendon, which can be reproduced by rolling the tendon under the examiner's thumb or with resisted flexion of the elbow.

tion of the diagnosis. Acute tears usually are treated surgically in younger, active patients. Long-standing tendon rupture usually is not painful and may not require attention.

Adhesive Capsulitis

Adhesive capsulitis is a perplexing syndrome associated with pain and limited motion of the shoulder. The shoulder capsule is thickened and may be adherent, and the volume of the joint is dramatically decreased. A number of associations have been noted, including prior injury or trauma to the shoulder or chest wall, which may limit shoulder motion; however, a number of other factors, including diabetes and thyroid disease, have been associated. Patients usually present with pain felt diffusely in the shoulder and experiencing limitation of motion. Over several months, pain tends to resolve, but motion may be progressively limited. This phase generated the term "frozen shoulder." Many patients will have "thawing" of the shoulder over the next year or two with return of motion. Prevention is the obvious initial aim of therapy. Range of motion exercises are prescribed for individuals with illnesses which limit shoulder motion. In those with symptoms, intra-articular injections are helpful in alleviating pain and allowing more comfortable range of motion exercises. Often, injections composed of corticosteroids and several milliliters of lidocaine are administered. In the past, manipulation under general anesthesia has been recommended. This is rarely necessary and has been associated with complications, including fracture of the humerus. Additionally, post-operative pain often limits range of motion, thus prolonging symptoms.

Reflex Sympathetic Dystrophy Syndrome

Reflex sympathetic dystrophy syndrome (RSDS) has been recognized since the Civil War, and historically has been known by a number of eponyms, including shoulder-hand syndrome, algodystrophy, and Sudeck's dystrophy. Considerable speculation has led to the hypothesis that, whatever the initiating events, reflex neurological events lead to vasospasm and other autonomic-appearing changes responsible for the syndrome. Initial descriptions have linked RSDS with chest trauma, but cerebrovascular disorders, myocardial infarctions, and pneumonia have been associated with the development of RSDS. Although, this syndrome may be seen in the lower extremity, it is most often recognized in the arm. Clinically, RSDS is characterized by:

- Pain
- Puffy and diffuse swelling of the hand
- Vasomotor instability.

The pain is often described as diffuse and burning in character. The shoulder and the hand may be diffusely tender and the hand may be swollen. Diffuse sweating may be noted in the hand, which may be associated with either vasodilatation or vasoconstriction. This phase of the syndrome may last for up to 6 months, to be followed by a dystrophic phase characterized by skin thickening. A final phase may occur where there is atrophy and contracture development. Not all patients diagnosed with RSDS will report that all phases have been present.

The diagnosis of RSDS is usually made clinically; however, later in the course, plain radiographs of the hand may reveal a patchy osteoporosis. Further bone scans generally demonstrate increased and persistent uptake diffusely in the hand. Therapeutically, pain relief and exercise of the extremity are the cornerstones of therapy. A number of other interventions have been tried with variable success. In resistant cases, a brief course of corticosteroids may be of use. Sympathetic block has been advocated by some; usually, multiple blocks are required and, even then, success rates are low.

Thoracic Outlet Syndrome

Thoracic outlet syndrome is compression of the neurovascular structures in one of three anatomic areas, as they exit the neck (Figure 17.6). The first is between the scalene muscles, where the brachial plexus leaves the neck and the subclavian artery exits the thorax. Variations in the muscle attachments or a cervical rib may compress this vessel or the plexus. The second is behind the clavicle, where the plexus and both the subclavian artery and vein run. Anomalies of the clavicle, eg, after a fracture or compression due to wearing back packs or brassiere straps,

FIGURE 17.6 — THORACIC OUTLET SYNDROME

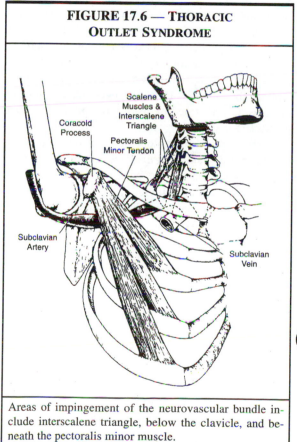

Areas of impingement of the neurovascular bundle include interscalene triangle, below the clavicle, and beneath the pectoralis minor muscle.

17

may occur causing symptoms. Last, the vessels and the brachial plexus run beneath the pectoralis muscle and compression may occur when the shoulder is abducted and externally rotated. Those who sleep or work with their hand in that position may have symptoms.

The symptoms of thoracic outlet syndrome are dependent upon the specific structure that is compressed. Plexus compression may lead to paresthesia, particularly in a C8 to T1 distribution, or even weakness and atrophy. Vascular compression can lead to edema or ischemic changes. A number of clinical maneuvers have been devised as attempts to determine if there is vascular compression in the neck. Adson's test, which is thought to determine if there is compression of the subclavian artery between the scalene muscles, is performed by asking the patient to rotate the neck as a Valsalva maneuver is performed. A positive test is the development of symptoms and a decreased pulse. Taking an exaggerated military stance, with the shoulders pulled back and down, tests the capacity of the retroclavicular space. The hyperabduction test is accomplished by feeling the radial pulse as the arm is abducted to 90 degrees (and externally rotated) and is thought to detect compression beneath the pectoralis minor.

Historically, thoracic outlet syndrome has been an overdiagnosed condition and many cervical ribs (occurring in nearly 1% of the population) have been deposited in pathology departments without producing any clinical improvement. A careful evaluation where symptoms and clinical findings are concordant is most likely to yield a correct diagnosis. Generally, when symptoms are intermittent, changes in activities may lead to symptomatic improvement. It is the rare patient who would need to be subjected to surgical intervention.

A number of conditions that cause pain around the pelvis are frequently interpreted as hip disease and should be considered in patients who have arthritis of the hip that does not appear to be responding appropriately. Hip arthritis is perceived as pain in the:

- Groin
- Buttock
- Referred pain to the knee.

Pain radiating from the back may be perceived in the buttock and confused with hip pain. Of course, hip motion will not reproduce symptoms due to back pain. Bursal pain is also a frequent consideration when there is pain around the pelvis (Figure 17.7). Pain due to trochanteric bursitis (the bursa over the greater femoral trochanter at the gluteal insertion sites) is felt laterally and patients often note that they have pain at

FIGURE 17.7 — BURSAL PAIN AROUND PELVIS

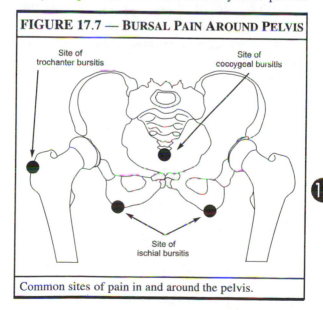

Site of
trochanter bursitis

Site of
cocoygeal bursitis

Site of
ischial bursitis

Common sites of pain in and around the pelvis.

17

night when they attempt to sleep on that side. Palpation over the area reproduces pain, and it is rapidly relieved by local injections of lidocaine and depot corticosteroids.

Ischial bursitis is a consideration when patients note localized pain while sitting. This bursa, which separates the ischium from the gluteus maximus, may become inflamed after local trauma. Again, local steroid injections are usually helpful. Other bursa around the hip and pelvis rarely are symptomatic.

Knee

In addition to arthritis, knee pain may be either derived from lesions in bursa or tendons or due to mechanical derangement (Figure 17.8). The latter, is often preceded by a memorable traumatic event. Meniscal tears may be suggested by joint space tenderness and the McMurray or Apley grind tests. Collateral ligament lesions are suggested by instability noted when the knee is flexed to about 30 degrees.

Anterior knee pain may also have several sources. Arthritis involving the patellofemoral joint is suspected when there is pain and crepitus with knee flexion and increased discomfort with activities that stress this joint, such as transversing stairs. Malalignment of the patella, with increased lateral motion of the patella relative to its proximal motion during knee flexion, may respond to quadricep strengthening exercises and stretching of the iliotibial band. Rarely, patella realignment may be indicated. Pain due to prepatellar bursitis is felt anteriorly in the knee and at the lower patella or over the patellar tendon. This may be precipitated by excessive kneeling.

Osgood-Schlatter disease is seen in children as pain at the insertion site of the patellar tendon into the tibial tubercle. Symptoms usually respond to analgesics such as acetaminophen or NSAIDs and time.

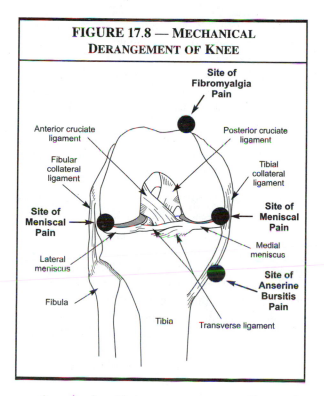

FIGURE 17.8 — MECHANICAL DERANGEMENT OF KNEE

Site of Fibromyalgia Pain

Anterior cruciate ligament

Posterior cruciate ligament

Fibular collateral ligament

Tibial collateral ligament

Site of Meniscal Pain

Site of Meniscal Pain

Medial meniscus

Lateral meniscus

Site of Anserine Bursitis Pain

Fibula

Tibia

Transverse ligament

Anserine bursitis is a common cause of knee pain and is frequently seen in patients with osteoarthritis or other forms of arthritis in which there is a valgus deformity of the knee. Pain is felt medially and reproduced by pressure over the bursa, which is located medially just below the joint space near the sartorius insertion site. Patients often note that pain is worse at night when they lie on their side with the knees together. Another bursa, the "no-name" bursa, is also located medially in the knee, anterior to the medial collateral ligament. Bursitis is often remedied by local steroid injections. Misalignment of the knee with a valgus deformity may cause recurrent anserine bursitis and may be difficult to treat. Strengthening exercises may help. If the valgus deformity is due to a preexisting arthritis, it may continue to recur.

A popliteal, colloquially known as the Baker's, cyst is herniation of the posterior aspect of the knee capsule into the popliteal space. The diagnosis is generally made on physical examination, but may be confirmed by ultrasonography. Should the cyst rupture, it may track down the back of the leg and simulate a deep venous thrombosis. Obviously, anticoagulation is not useful, and may be harmful in this setting.

Ankle and Foot

Despite the complexity of the structures in the foot, a careful examination usually will uncover causes of ankle and foot pain (Figure 17.9). Achilles tendinitis, in addition to being seen in the seronegative spondyloarthropathies, may occur in isolation after overuse or due to trauma (including trauma due to poorly fitting shoes). Pain is localized to the insertion site in the calcaneus. The retrocalcaneal bursa lies deep to the Achilles tendon proximate to its insertion site and when inflamed, differentiation from Achilles tendinitis may be impossible. Rest, NSAIDs and a heel cup to help unload the tendon is often useful in both conditions. Many physicians feel definite reluctance toward injection of this tendon, as it is heavily loaded and when inflamed, may be more likely to rupture.

Posterior tibial tendinitis is perceived as pain posterior to the medial malleolus, which is worsened by passive eversion of the ankle or resisted inversion. Palpation over this area will generally reproduce pain and relief can be gained by rest, NSAIDs and injections. Tendinitis of the flexor hallucis longus also may be perceived behind the medial malleolus, which in addition may impair flexion of the great toe.

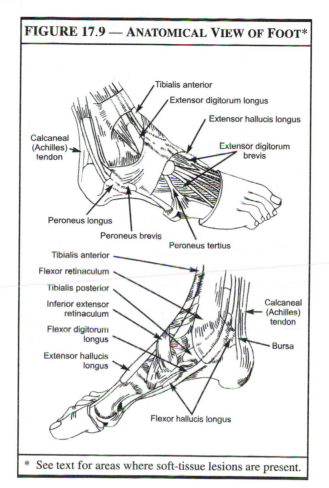

FIGURE 17.9 — ANATOMICAL VIEW OF FOOT*

Tibialis anterior

Extensor digitorum longus

Extensor hallucis longus

Extensor digitorum brevis

Calcaneal (Achilles) tendon

Peroneus longus

Peroneus brevis

Peroneus tertius

Tibialis anterior

Flexor retinaculum

Tibialis posterior

Inferior extensor retinaculum

Flexor digitorum longus

Extensor hallucis longus

Calcaneal (Achilles) tendon

Bursa

Flexor hallucis longus

* See text for areas where soft-tissue lesions are present.

Plantar fasciitis is generally felt as pain at the insertion site of the fascia into the calcaneus. Trauma, overuse, or poorly supporting shoes may lead to inflammation and pain often described as burning, which is worse after beginning ambulation. Symptoms usually respond to rest, shoe support or orthotics, and NSAIDs. Occasionally, when other treatments fail, steroid injections may be useful.

17

Tarsal tunnel syndrome is compression of the posterior tibial nerve behind and below the medial malleolus by the local retinaculum. It may develop in conjunction with ankle arthritis, trauma, or ankle deformity. Pain, which is described as burning in character, may be present along with paresthesia or numbness over the medial foot and sole. Weakness of flexion of the great toe may also be observed. Rest and local injections are often helpful, but decompression may be necessary. Electrodiagnostic studies can be helpful, particularly when the diagnosis is in doubt prior to surgery.

Morton's neuroma may develop between the toes, most often the third and fourth. Compression of the interdigital nerve may lead to burning paresthesia in the toe. Rest and local injections are helpful. Occasionally, excision is necessary.

SUGGESTED READING

Bovim G, Schrader H, Sand T. Neck pain in the general population. *Spine*. 1994;19:1307-1309.

Hollingsworth GR, Ellis RM, Hattersley TS. Comparison of injection techniques for shoulder pain: results of a double blind randomised study. *Br Med J*. 1983;287:1339-1341.

The ankle and foot. In: Sheon RP, Moskowitz RW, Goldberg VM, eds. *Soft Tissue Rheumatic Pain: Recognition, Management and Prevention*. 3rd ed. Baltimore, Md: Williams & Wilkins; 1996;Chapter 12:243-266.

The knee. In: Sheon RP, Moskowitz RW, Goldberg VM, eds. *Soft Tissue Rheumatic Pain: Recognition, Management and Prevention*. 3rd ed. Baltimore, Md: Williams & Wilkins; 1996;Chapter 10:217-236.

Steinbrocker O, Aryros TG. Frozen shoulder: treatment by local injections of depot corticosteroids. *Arch Phys Med Rehabil*. 1974; 55:209-213.

18 Systemic Lupus Erythematosus

Systemic lupus erythematosus (SLE) is the prototypical disorder mentioned when autoimmune diseases are discussed. Protean in its presentation, its clinical manifestations can vary from a mild rash together with a nonerosive arthritis to a life-threatening illness with involvement of the brain and kidneys.

Pathogenesis

Most theories regarding the pathogenesis of SLE begin with recognition that a particular genetic predisposition is necessary. Monozygotic twins are concordant for SLE much more often than dizygotic twins, indicating a significant genetic influence and leading to suggestions that environmental exposure plays no role in its development. Consistent with this conclusion are observations from the murine lupus model; the MRL lpr/lpr mouse develops lupus even in germ-free environments. Studies directed at identifying specific genes or gene loci linked to SLE risk, have established that class II human leukocyte antigens (HLAs) DR2 and DR3 afford an approximately threefold risk. Further studies have expanded on and confirmed these observations. The presence of these antigens may allow for the persistence and expansion of T clones that are autoreactive, thus paving the way for humoral and cellular responses.

However, a number of other genes have been linked to the development of lupus. Included among these are the complement proteins C4 and C2, in which homozygous deficiency is a strong risk factor for SLE. Polymorphisms of tumor necrosis factor (TNF)-α and Fc receptor genes or promoters also are risk factors and may influence the inflammatory response or the clearance of immune complexes. Ultimately, there is development of a humoral and cellular inflammatory response targeted to certain organs that leads to the clinical expression of the disease.

Occurrence

Systemic lupus erythematosus is not an uncommon disorder and it has definite racial and gender predilections. Overall, lupus is seen much more often in women, in some series representing 80% to 90% of the cases. Interestingly, when the onset is in older individuals, the gender difference narrows considerably. Blacks develop lupus much more commonly than whites.

Systemic lupus erythematosus is relatively common in the general population. Older studies placed the prevalence of lupus at between 14.6 to 50.7 per 100,000 population, but the study representing the low end of this range was performed prior to the establishment of criteria for SLE. Also, early studies have often been based on patients presenting to medical centers and particularly to subspecialists such as rheumatologists. By their nature, these studies again tended to underestimate the prevalence of SLE. As knowledge has evolved, the diagnosis of SLE has become more common, and treatment is frequently in the hands of primary-care physicians.

Approximately 90% of patients with SLE are women. Further, blacks develop SLE more commonly than whites. For example, Fessel, who found that SLE occurred in 50.7 per 100,000 population, also concluded that the prevalence rates are 143 per 100,000 in all women and 408 per 100,000 in black women.

Other studies have confirmed the greater prevalence of SLE in black women.

Further, contemporary and relevant information suggests that older data underestimate the true prevalence of SLE. Hochberg and colleagues surveyed the population by randomly dialing households and found that, among women, the prevalence of self-reported, physician-diagnosed SLE was 454 cases per 100,000. Based upon these data, Hochberg et al concluded that they could be 95% confident that the self-reported prevalence of SLE among white women would be between 254 and 750 cases per 100,000. Further studies have shed more light on the issue of the prevalence of SLE. Hennekens et al surveyed 384,713 women and found that 1 out of 246 reported that they had lupus, while Johnson et al found 200 cases per 100,000 women when surveying a community for previously undiagnosed cases of SLE.

Clinical Features

Essentially any organ system may be affected by SLE, though it is particular combinations of signs which allow for the correct diagnosis and differentiation from other disorders. Utilization of criteria developed in conjunction with the American College of Rheumatology provide excellent sensitivity and specificity (Table 18.1).

Despite the importance of involvement of other systems, mucocutaneous involvement is the hallmark of SLE. The malar or "butterfly" rash is an area of erythema over the malar aspect of the face (Figure 18.1). Typically, this lesion is:

- Raised
- Fixed
- Erythematous
- Sometimes painful

18

TABLE 18.1 — 1982 REVISED CRITERIA FOR CLASSIFICATION OF SYSTEMIC LUPUS ERYTHEMATOSUS

Criterion	Definition
Malar rash	Fixed erythema, flat or raised, over the malar eminences, tending to spare the nasolabial folds
Discoid rash	Erythematous raised patches with adherent keratotic scaling and follicular plugging; atrophic scarring may occur in older lesions
Photosensitivity	Skin rash as a result of unusual reaction to sunlight, by patient history or physician observation
Oral ulcers	Oral or nasopharyngeal ulceration, usually painless, observed by a physician
Arthritis	Nonerosive arthritis involving two or more peripheral joints, characterized by tenderness, swelling, or effusion
Serositis	Pleuritis—convincing history of pleuritic pain or rub heard by a physician or evidence of pleural effusion OR Pericarditis—documented by ECG or rub or evidence of pericardial effusion

Criterion	Definition
Renal disorder	Persistent proteinuria > 0.5 g/d or > 3+ if quantitation not performed OR Cellular casts—may be red cell, hemoglobin, granular, tubular or mixed
Neurologic disorder	Seizures—in the absence of offending drugs or known metabolic derangements, eg, uremia, ketoacidosis or electrolyte imbalance OR Psychosis—in the absence of offending drugs or known metabolic derangements, eg, uremia, ketoacidosis or electrolyte imbalance
Hematologic disorder	Hemolytic anemia—with reticulocytosis OR Leukopenia—less than 4000/mm³ total on two or more ccasions OR Lymphopenia—less than 1500/mm³ on two or more occasions OR Thrombocytopenia—less than 100,000/mm³ in the absence of offending drugs

Continued

Immunologic disorder	Positive lupus erythematosus cell preparation OR Anti-DNA: antibody to native DNA in abnormal titer OR Anti-Sm: presence of antibody to Sm nuclear antigen OR False-positive serologic test for syphilis known to be positive for at least 6 months and confirmed by *Treponema pallidum* immobilization or fluorescent treponemal antibody absorption test
Antinuclear antibody	An abnormal titer of antinuclear antibody by immunofluorescence or an equivalent assay at any point in time and in the absence of drugs known to be associated with "drug-induced lupus" syndrome

* The proposed classification is based on 11 criteria. For the purpose of identifying patients in clinical studies, a person shall be said to have systemic lupus erythematosus if any four or more of the 11 criteria are present, serially or simultaneously, during any interval of observation.

Tan EM, et al. *Arthritis Rheum.* 1982;25:1271-1277.

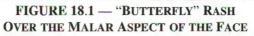

FIGURE 18.1 — "BUTTERFLY" RASH OVER THE MALAR ASPECT OF THE FACE

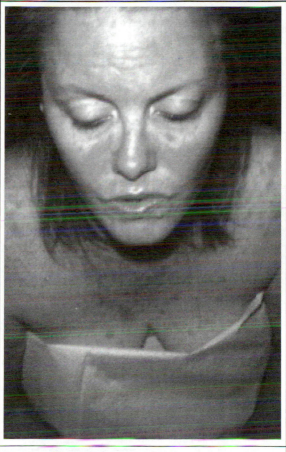

Courtesy of Syntex Laboratories, Inc.

- Usually symmetric
- Sparing of the nasolabial fold.

Discoid lupus erythematosus (DLE) is a scaly erythematous plaque-like lesion which can be present anywhere, but is often seen on the face and scalp (Figure 18.2). Careful examination of the lesion reveals:
- Areas of follicular plugging
- Telangiectasia
- Skin atrophy.

FIGURE 18.2 — DISCOID LUPUS ERYTHEMATOSUS OF THE FACE

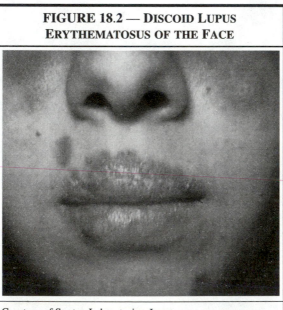

Courtesy of Syntex Laboratories, Inc.

These lesions may heal with scarring and hyper- or hypopigmentation. When these lesions occur in the scalp, they may be associated with patchy, but permanent, hair loss. Of course, DLE may occur in isolation and is not necessarily indicative of systemic disease.

About one third of patients with SLE report development of a rash with sun exposure. Typically, this is an unusual persistent erythema which occurs with minimal sun exposure and must be differentiated from the normal erythema induced by exposure to ultraviolet radiation. A patient spontaneously reporting a change with sun exposure is often more informative than a questionable sun response elicited from in-depth questioning.

In addition to the skin lesions discussed above, a number of other, more nonspecific lesions are sometimes seen in patients with SLE, such as:

- Livedo reticularis
- Petechiae
- Urticaria.

Subacute cutaneous lupus erythematosus (SCLE) is an erythematous rash, usually in sun-exposed areas, best recognized as serpiginous, annular plaques, frequently with a relative central clearing. SCLE may also appear as psoriaform lesions or small macules. This lesion is not indicative of SLE, as only about half of patients with SCLE have both.

Careful examination of oral, nasal or vaginal mucosa may reveal ulcers. They are usually well demarcated with an erythematous base (Figure 18.3). Frequently, these are not painful.

Arthritis is common in patients with lupus. On occasion, it may present with deformities reminiscent of rheumatoid arthritis (RA), with ulnar drift at the metacarpophalangeal and swan neck or boutonnière's deformities. In contrast to RA, the arthritis of lupus is nonerosive and the deformities are correctable. In most individuals, the arthritis is a symmetrical polyarthritis with particular involvement of the small joints of the hands, wrists and knees.

Serosal inflammation in SLE may involve the pleural, pericardial or abdominal serosa. Pleural in-

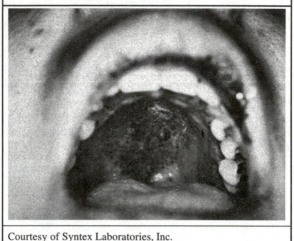
volvement is the most common and the clinical manifestations can vary from severe and typical pleuritic pain to asymptomatic pleural effusions. In most individuals, effusions are small, but occasionally they can occupy much of the thoracic cavity. Pleural effusions are often seen in the context of active lupus elsewhere. Fluid is usually exudative and lupus erythematosus (LE) cells may be found. Less often patients with SLE may develop interstitial lung disease, initially detected as a decreased diffusing capacity. Most often this is a chronic process, but some present acutely. A rare patient will present with diffuse pulmonary hemorrhage which, despite vigorous supportive care, is often fatal.

In addition to pericarditis, coronary arteritis, myocarditis, and Libman-Sacks endocarditis are all features of lupus cardiac involvement. Arteritis and myocarditis are somewhat unusual, but more often patients with lupus develop atherosclerotic coronary disease.

In addition to routine risk factors, patients with lupus have hypertension, and the inflammatory process and corticosteroids have a deleterious effect on lipids.

Renal involvement in SLE may take a number of forms. The glomerular disease is often asymptomatic early in the course, and the only evidence may be an abnormal urinalysis or perhaps an elevation of blood pressure. Classification of lupus nephritis has been standardized according to the World Health Organization (Table 18.2). Further, a chronicity and activity index has been developed which is sometimes used to manage the renal disease (Table 18.2).

Rare patients with lupus develop a frank psychosis or seizures. This is usually in the setting of obviously active disease with fevers, altered mental status, and seizures. Untreated, coma and death may ensue. In this setting, examination of the spinal fluid is usually abnormal, but nonspecifically so, with elevation of protein and mild increases in white blood cells (WBCs). A number of other central nervous system (CNS) syndromes have been associated with lupus, including chorea and stroke syndromes. CNS thrombotic episodes have been attributed to the presence of anti-phospholipid antibodies. More often, more subtle neuropsychological changes are attributed to SLE. These include cognitive impairment and headaches. In some, differentiating these from the myriad of other causes, including anxiety, may be difficult.

Laboratory Tests and Radiographs

Perhaps more so with SLE than with any other rheumatic disorder, results of laboratory tests are an essential feature of diagnosis and management, but are also frequently misused, leading to unnecessary expense and patient anxiety.

18

TABLE 18.2 — RENAL PATHOLOGY SCORING SYSTEM*

Activity Index	Chronicity Index
Glomerular Abnormalities	
1. Cellular proliferation	1. Glomerular sclerosis
2. Fibrinoid necrosis, karyorrhexis	2. Fibrous crescents
3. Cellular crescents	
4. Hyaline thrombi, wire loops	
5. Leukocyte infiltration	
Tubulointerstitial Abnormalities	
1. Mononuclear-cell infiltration	1. Interstitial fibrosis
	2. Tubular atrophy

* Fibrinoid necrosis and cellular crescents are weighted by a factor of 2. Maximum score of activity index is 24; chronicity index is 12.

Serological testing is the best example. Antinuclear antibodies (ANAs) are found in serum of essentially all patients with SLE. However, ANA detection is not indicative of SLE or, for that matter, disease at all. Several studies have now demonstrated that approximately 30% of normal women will have detectable ANA in their serum. As a group, patients with SLE tend to have higher titers of these antibodies, but there is broad overlap. Moreover, there is no evidence to indicate that in an individual patient, following titers is useful in prognosis. Patterns of ANA (speckled, homogeneous, rim, nucleolar and cytoplasmic) have been described and reflect the specific ANA subsets.

Analysis of autoantibodies has become much more sophisticated and many ANA determinants have been found. Some of them are useful diagnostically and may also select groups more likely to experience certain complications of SLE. Anti-double-stranded (ds) DNA antibodies are found in about one third of patients with SLE, particularly in those who may develop nephritis. In a general sense, titers of dsDNA antibodies reflect disease activity, but there are many exceptions. When detected on tissue substrates, they generally appear as a homogeneous or rim pattern. Except for low titers, these antibodies are rarely seen in other disorders or in normals. Presence of this antibody is considered as fulfilling one of the diagnostic criteria for SLE.

Antibodies to Sm bind to the RNA-protein complex responsible for removing introns to form mRNA. In tissue preparations, anti-Sm appears in a speckled pattern. The presence or titer of this antibody does not correlate with disease activity.

Other antibodies may detect groups of SLE patients with certain clinical characteristics. In most, the clinical presentation is more important than the presence of an antibody. Anti-SSA (previously Ro) anti-

18

bodies is also seen in about one third of SLE patients, particularly in those who have sun sensitivity, sicca symptoms, and lymphopenia. Moreover, these antibodies are detected in infants with neonatal lupus and have been found to bind to the infants' conducting systems and are responsible for cases of congenital heart block. Anti-SSB (previously La) is often seen in conjunction with SSA and seems to be present in patients who do not develop nephritis. Antiphospholipid antibodies are responsible for the false-positive syphilis serology. In these patients, the fluorescent treponeme antibody is negative. These antibodies are often, but not always, responsible for the prolongation of the partial thromboplastin time (PTT) frequently seen in SLE patients. Often, these antibodies will be detected without a clear clinical correlate, but they have been linked to thrombotic episodes, recurrent abortions, and Libman-Sacks endocarditis. Antiribosomal P protein antibodies have been disputably linked to psychosis.

Levels of complement proteins may vary considerably in patients with lupus. In those with active disease with limited consumption of complement proteins, CH50, C4, and C2 may actually be elevated. Alternatively, in many patients with active renal disease, levels may drop, indicating either consumption or perhaps detecting the patient with a hereditary deficiency. Like dsDNA antibodies, decreasing levels of complement components may predict worsening disease in particular individuals. Again, there are enough exceptions that placing full reliance on levels is not prudent.

Leukopenia is often seen and its observation is diagnostically useful, particularly when it cannot be attributed to medications. Analysis of the differential usually demonstrates a lymphopenia; neutropenia is unusual, but often there is an eosinophilia. Elevation of WBC counts may reflect steroid use or, more ominously, an intercurrent infection.

Anemia is seen in most patients with lupus. Often, it is due to either chronic disease or iron deficiency related to therapy or menstruation. Autoimmune hemolytic anemia is seen less often, and is usually associated with a positive Coomb's test. Signs of hemolysis are seen when blood smears are examined or are indicated by elevated LDH and reticulocyte counts, and low haptoglobins.

Thrombocytopenia may be a manifestation of idiopathic thrombocytopenic purpura, which can occur in isolation long before the diagnosis of lupus is made. Rarely, a syndrome of fever, mental status changes, renal dysfunction, thrombocytopenia, and hemolysis consistent with thrombotic thrombocytopenia purpura may be seen in patients with lupus.

Other laboratory abnormalities may be reflective of lupus involvement of a particular organ. A urinalysis, serum chemistries, and test of creatine kinase levels may be useful in evaluating and following patients with SLE.

Radiographs similarly may be useful in evaluating or following patients with SLE. Joint radiographs may reveal some cartilage loss and deformity, but erosions are not part of SLE. Although a syndrome of erosive arthritis in a patient with SLE has been termed rhupus, perhaps simply a coincidental occurrence of SLE and RA in the same patient. Chest radiographs or ultrasound studies may be helpful when serositis or interstitial lung disease is suspected.

Diagnosis

18

The American College of Rheumatology has established diagnostic criteria for SLE. Although these criteria were put forth so that there would be some clinical uniformity for studies, they have been largely employed in clinical settings. An occasional patient with SLE will not fulfill the diagnostic criteria and an occasional patient without SLE will.

Most of the diagnostic criteria are self-explanatory. As noted, the malar rash is fixed and should not be confused with similar-appearing disorders such as seborrhea. Photosensitivity should be an unusual reaction to sun, not simply a predictable sun burn. Oral ulcers should be differentiated from those of viral origin. Arthritis should not be confused with tenderness from periarticular points, as is often seen in fibromyalgia. Chest pain should be reliably attributed to serosal inflammation prior to considering this a fulfilling diagnostic criterion. The numerous conditions which cause pain (including chest wall pain) should be excluded.

Patients with fibromyalgia, who also have an ANA, are sometimes confused with SLE; generally, a careful examination differentiates the two. Early RA (prior to the development of erosions), dermatomyositis, scleroderma and other inflammatory rheumatic disease may be difficult to differentiate from SLE. Profound thyroid disease may present with joint and muscle pain, cardiac symptoms, and an ANA. An occasional patient with lymphoma will have evidence of serosal involvement, joint pain, abnormal blood counts, and an ANA. Differentiation is usually made by biopsy.

Management

Treatment of patients with lupus is often complex and challenging. In most patients, avoidance of sun exposure by using sun screens, wide-brim hats, and long sleeved shirts is prescribed. Other therapies, in most instances, must be tailored to the individual patient. Careful weighing of the sign or symptom being treated and how they are to be objectively evalu-
252

ated, and the potential risk of therapy, must be considered to avoid unnecessary therapeutic complications. As with therapy for all rheumatic diseases, attention should be given to general health-care maintenance. Vaccinations should be brought up to date, blood pressure and blood sugars should be controlled, and electrolytes and fluid balance maintained.

Nonsteroidal anti-inflammatory drugs (NSAIDs) are frequently useful in treating arthritis and occasionally the serositis seen in SLE. In those with renal involvement or risk of gastrointestinal complications, NSAIDs may need to be discontinued.

Antimalarials, such as hydroxychloroquine and others, are useful in patients who have relatively mild lupus or as steroid-sparing agents. Joint pain, skin rashes, fatigue, serositis, and even thrombocytopenia may respond to these agents.

Corticosteroids are, at times, used as therapy for many facets of the disease. In general, high doses are reserved for life-threatening complications, such as severe thrombocytopenia or autoimmune hemolytic anemia, CNS vasculitis, aggressive renal disease, or pneumonitis. Doses of 1 mg/kg/d of prednisone are usually used. In extremely active disease, divided daily doses may be more effective. More moderate doses of steroids are usually sufficient to treat serosal inflammation. Therapy should be guided by objective measures and by each patient's response to therapy, if at all possible. In most situations, steroid tapering should not be halted based solely on subjective symptoms. Further, many patients will develop myalgias or arthralgias simply related to steroid tapering. The risk of long-term, high-dose corticosteroids is considerable and every attempt should be made to minimize their use.

Other agents are used in certain situations. Azathioprine is useful as a steroid-sparing agent and is used to treat nephritis and arthritis in particular. Meth-

18

otrexate, used as low-dose weekly pulse therapy, is useful for treating arthritis. Excretion of this drug is through the kidneys and care is necessary when there is renal dysfunction. Cyclophosphamide is often used in managing the disease of patients with proliferative glomerulonephritis. Used as a daily dose, success (as measured by not requiring dialysis) is superior to treatment with steroids alone. However, side effects, including hematocytopenias, malignancies, sterility, and hemorrhagic cystitis, are common. More recently, cyclophosphamide has been effectively administered as a monthly pulse (750 mg/m^2/mo) for about 6 months followed by doses every 2 or 3 months for about 2 years.

A combination of recognizing milder cases and careful attention to the details of management have led to remarkable improvement in the reported survival in SLE. Ten-year survival is now about 90%. Cardiovascular and renal complications and infections remain the leading causes of mortality.

SUGGESTED READING

Austin HA III, Klippel JH, Balow JE, et al. Therapy of lupus nephritis. Controlled trial of prednisone and cytotoxic drugs. *N Engl J Med*. 1986;314:614-619.

Austin HA III, Muenz LR, Joyce KM, et al. Prognostic factors in lupus nephritis. Contribution of renal histologic data. *Am J Med*. 1983;75:382-391.

Fessel WJ. Systemic lupus erythematosus in the community. Incidence, prevalence, outcome, and first symptoms; the high prevalence in black women. *Arch Intern Med*. 1974;134:1027-1035.

Gladman DD, Urowitz MB, Cole E, Ritchie S, Chang CH, Churg J. Kidney biopsy in SLE/ IA clinical-morphologic evaluation. *Quart J Med*. 1989;73: 1125-1153.

Hennekens CH, Lee IM, Cook NR, et al. Self-reported breast implants and connective-tissue diseases in female health professionals. A retrospective cohort study [published erratum appears in *JAMA*. 1998;279:198]. *JAMA*. 1996;275:616-621.

Hochberg M, Perlmutter DL, White B, pet al. The prevalence of self-reported, physician-diagnosed systemic lupus erythematosus. *Arthritis Rheum*. 1994;37(S):S-302.

Johnson AE, Gordon C, Hobbs FD, Bacon PA. Undiagnosed systemic lupus erythematosus in the community. *Lancet*. 1996;347: 367-369.

Tan EM, Cohen AS, Fries JF, et al. The 1982 revised criteria for the classification of systemic lupus erythematosus. *Arthritis Rheum*. 1982;25:1271-1277.

18

19 Vasculitis

Despite the simplicity of its definition (an inflammation of blood vessels), vasculitis, perhaps more than any other rheumatic disorder, is sometimes the source of considerable consternation to the clinician. The diagnosis can be difficult and, occasionally, the course catastrophic. A number of classification schemes have been proposed and may at times be useful when considering a patient with vasculitis. What follows is a brief clinical discussion of some of the more common forms of primary vasculitis. Of course, vasculitis may be seen with many of the inflammatory rheumatic diseases discussed elsewhere and will not be discussed further here. In addition, a number of other conditions, such as malignancies and certain infections, are at times associated with vasculitis and also will not be discussed here.

Takayasu's Arteritis

Affecting the aorta and its major branches, Takayasu's arteritis tends to be seen in young women, particularly those of Asian descent. Early symptoms may be vague, reflecting the systemic nature of the disease, including:

- Malaise
- Arthralgias
- Mylagias
- Fever (Table 19.1).

This may be followed in weeks or months with signs or symptoms due to vascular insufficiency. Alterna-

TABLE 19.1 — 1990 CRITERIA FOR THE CLASSIFICATION OF TAKAYASU ARTERITIS

Criterion	Definition
Age at disease onset ≤ 40 years	Development of symptoms or findings related to Takayasu arteritis at age ≤ 40 years
Claudication of extremities	Development and worsening of fatigue and discomfort in muscles of one or more extremity while in use, especially the upper extremities
Decreased brachial artery pulse	Decreased pulsation of one or both brachial arteries
Blood pressure difference > 10 mm Hg	Difference of > 10 mm Hg in systolic blood pressure between arms
Bruit over subclavian arteries or aorta	Bruit audible on auscultation over one or both subclavian arteries or abdominal aorta
Arteriogram abnormality	Arteriographic narrowing or occlusion of the entire aorta, its primary branches, or large arteries in the proximal upper or lower extremities, not due to arteriosclerosis, fibromuscular dysplasia, or similar causes; changes usually focal or segmental

* For purposes of classification, a patient shall be said to have Takayasu arteritis if at least three of these six criteria are present. The presence of any three or more criteria yields a sensitivity of 90.5% and a specificity of 97.8%.

Reprinted from: Arend WP, et al. *Arthritis Rheum.* 1990;33:1129-1134.

tively, vascular insufficiency may be the initial symptoms in some patients. Complaints may include:

- Headaches
- Dizziness
- Visual disturbances
- Limb claudication.

Absent pulses, bruits, or discrepancies between blood pressures in the contralateral limb are suggestive clinical findings. Cardiac involvement may be manifest as heart failure due to either:

- Hypertension (with renal artery involvement)
- Aortic regurgitation (due to dilatation of the aortic root)
- Coronary ischemia (due to direct involvement of the coronary arteries)
- Secondary to pulmonary artery hypertension.

Routine laboratory tests demonstrate nonspecific changes. Acute phase proteins are elevated. Chest radiographs may reveal widening of the aorta. In suggestive cases, either digital subtraction angiography or magnetic resonance angiography of the entire aorta and its major branches is usually diagnostic.

Initial treatment generally includes corticosteroids, typically with prednisone at doses of about 1 mg/kg/d. Systemic features resolve rapidly; pulses may return and symptoms due to ischemia may resolve. Some patients will be able to taper the steroids, whereas others will have a more tumultuous course with exacerbations limiting the attempts to taper corticosteroids. Medications such as methotrexate or cyclophosphamide may be useful in these situations, but side effects, including early ovarian failure, may be a significant concern. Other therapies include those reflecting good medical care; in particular, control of hypertension is important. Revascularization procedures may be critical for restoring blood supply. Timing is important, however, as a vessel involved with the vasculitic process may be more likely to restenose or dehisce.

Polyarteritis Nodosa

A disease of medium and small vessels, polyarteritis nodosa (PAN) reflects the histological appearance of transmural vasculitis. Essentially, any muscular artery may be involved, although those in the lung tend to be spared. The disorder may afflict individuals of any age, but middle-aged individuals more often, and particularly men. PAN has been associated with hepatitis B and C infections. Initial symptoms are often vague, but frequently include:

- Malaise
- Fatigue
- Fever
- Abdominal pain.

Renal artery involvement is the most common, but may be asymptomatic and only apparent based on the development of hypertension, evidence of renal dysfunction, or an abnormal urinalysis. Many patients with PAN will have neurological abnormalities, most often of the peripheral nervous system. Mononeuritis multiplex is more characteristic, but other sensory or motor neuropathies may be present. Distal involvement, such as with a wrist or foot drop, is more distinctive.

Diagnosis is most convincingly made based on angiography, where multiple small aneurysms are usually seen, especially when other disorders, such as amphetamine abuse and atrial myxomas (which can have similar angiographic appearances), have been ruled out. Diagnostic criteria have also been developed (Table 19.2).

Therapy is usually initiated with high-dose corticosteroids. Often, there is some urgency in starting therapy as catastrophic complications can abruptly occur. Response is generally rapid. Many physicians caring for patients with PAN will add cyclophosphamide as a steroid-sparing agent and for more rapid control. Evidence that the addition of this agent improves long-term survival is lacking.

Wegener's Granulomatosis

Wegener's granulomatosis is a necrotizing granulomatous vasculitis involving the upper and lower respiratory tract coupled with a necrotizing glomerulonephritis. This disorder is unusual, and occurs most commonly in white adults of middle age. Nonspecific complaints, including fever, arthralgias and myalgias, are common. Upper respiratory complaints are most commonly those of chronic, therapy-unresponsive sinusitis. Other manifestations of Wegener's granulomatosis include:

- Mucosal ulceration
- Tracheal irritation and stenosis
- Chronic otitis
- Eye disorders, excluding exophthalmos.

Pulmonary involvement may be silent or present with a cough, which may be either dry or productive of bloody sputum. Chest radiographs reveal nodules, which often cavitate.

In general, respiratory symptoms are noted prior to renal involvement. When there is such involvement, the urinary sediment may be abnormal, with hematuria, pyuria and cellular casts. If untreated, renal involvement can rapidly lead to renal failure.

Diagnostic criteria have been developed (Table 19.3). Since their development, it has been recognized that the detection of antineutrophil cytoplasmic anti-

TABLE 19.2 — 1990 CRITERIA FOR THE CLASSIFICATION OF POLYARTERITIS NODOSA*

Criterion	Definition
Weight loss ≤ 4 kg	Loss of 4 kg or more of body weight since illness began, not due to dieting or other factors
Livedo reticularis	Mottled reticular pattern over the skin on portions of the extremities or torso
Testicular pain or tenderness	Pain or tenderness of the testicles, not due to infection, trauma or other causes
Myalgias, weakness, or leg tenderness	Diffuse myalgias, excluding shoulder and hip girdle, weakness of muscles, or tenderness of leg muscles
Mononeuropathy or polyneuropathy	Development of mononeuropathy, multiple mononeuropathies, or polyneuropathy
Diastolic BP > 90 mm Hg	Development of hypertension with the diastolic BP higher than 90 mm Hg
Elevated BUN or creatinine	Elevation of BUN > 40 mg/dL or creatinine > 1.5 mg/dL, not due to dehydration or obstruction

Hepatitis B virus	Presence of hepatitis B surface antigen or antibody in serum
Arteriographic abnormality	Arteriogram showing aneurysms or occlusions of the visceral arteries, not due to arteriosclerosis, fibromuscular dysplasia, or other noninflammatory causes
Biopsy of small- or medium-sized artery containing PMN	Histologic changes showing the presence of granulocytes or granulocytes and mononuclear leukocytes in the artery wall

Abbreviations: BP, blood pressure; BUN, blood urea nitrogen; PMN, polymorphonuclear neutrophils.

* For classification purposes, a patient shall be said to have polyarteritis nodosa if at least three of these 10 criteria are present. The presence of any three or more criteria yields a sensitivity of 82.2% and a specificity of 86.6%.

Reprinted from: Lightfoot RW Jr, et al. *Arthritis Rheum.* 1990;33:1091.

19

TABLE 19.3 — 1990 CRITERIA FOR THE CLASSIFICATION OF WEGENER'S GRANULOMATOSIS*

Criterion	Definition
Nasal or oral inflammation	Development of painful or painless oral ulcers or purulent or bloody nasal discharge
Abnormal chest radiograph	Chest radiograph showing the presence of nodules, fixed infiltrates, or cavities
Urinary sediment	Microhematuria (> 5 red blood cells per high-power field) or red cell casts in urine sediment
Granulomatous inflammation on biopsy	Histologic changes showing granulomatous inflammation within the wall of an artery or in the perivascular or extravascular area (artery or arteriole)

* For purposes of classification, a patient shall be said to have Wegener's granulomatosis if at least two of these four criteria are present. The presence of any two or more criteria yields a sensitivity of 88.2% and a specificity of 92.0%.

Reprinted from: Leavitt RY, et al. *Arthritis Rheum.* 1990;33:1101-1107.

bodies (ANCA), particularly those considered cANCA (in contradistinction to those that are perinuclear pANCA), is common in Wegener's. Although controversial, there has been a suggestion that cANCA titers reflect disease activity and may disappear when the disease is quiescent. Histologic confirmation of Wegener's granulomatosus is generally made on a biopsy of the respiratory tract. If the only apparent involvement is the lung, open lung biopsies may be necessary to obtain sufficient tissue. Characteristic changes include granulomas in a vessel or in the perivascular area. Renal findings are less specific and may simply demonstrate a focal and segmental glomerulonephritis.

Therapy is with both prednisone and cyclophosphamide, as this combination has been shown to improve survival when compared to treatment with steroids alone. Initially, cyclosphosphamide is given at doses of about 2/mg/kg/d and the dose adjusted until the white blood count is between about 3000 to 3500 cells/mm^3. After a year of therapy with remission induction, therapy is tapered. Prednisone is often given at doses of about 1 mg/kg/d for approximately a month. Thereafter, the dose is converted to alternate-day therapy and tapering off over about 6 months.

There has been ongoing interest in the role of trimethoprim/sulfamethoxazole in treating Wegener's. In most of the successful anecdotal reports, disease has been limited.

Churg-Strauss Vasculitis

Churg-Strauss vasculitis is a clinical syndrome composed of asthma, pulmonary infiltrates, eosinophilia, and peripheral medium- or small-vessel vasculitis. This often occurs sequentially, but may present together. Criteria have been put forth by the American College of Rheumatology (Table 19.4). Renal in-

19

TABLE 19.4 — 1990 CRITERIA FOR THE CLASSIFICATION OF CHURG-STRAUSS SYNDROME

Criterion	Definition
Asthma	History of wheezing or diffuse high-pitched rales on expiration
Eosinophilia	Eosinophilia > 10% on white blood cell differential count
History of allergy*	History of seasonal allergy (eg, allergic rhinitis) or other documented allergies, including food, contactants and others, *except* for drug allergy
Mononeuropathy or polyneuropathy	Development of mononeuropathy, multiple mononeuropathies, or polyneuropathy (ie, glove and stocking distribution) attributable to a systemic vasculitis
Pulmonary infiltrates, nonfixed	Migratory or transitory pulmonary infiltrates on radiographs (not including fixed infiltrates), attributable to a systemic vasculitis
Paranasal sinus abnormality	History of acute or chronic paranasal sinus pain or tenderness or radiographic opacification of the paranasal sinuses
Extravascular eosinophils	Biopsy, including artery, arteriole or venule, showing accumulations of eosinophils in extravascular areas

* History of allergy, other than asthma or drug-related, is included only in the tree classification criteria set and not in the traditional format criteria set, which requires four or more of the six other items listed here (and in Table 18.2).

Reprinted from: Masi AT, et al. *Arthritis Rheum.* 1990;33:1098.

volvement is distinctly unusual in Churg-Strauss, and the pulmonary involvement separates it from polyarteritis nodosa. The pulmonary lesions are infiltrates or nodules, which do not cavitate. Most patients respond promptly to high doses of corticosteroids, but those with resistant disease may benefit from the addition of azathioprine or cyclophosphamide.

Mucocutaneous Lymph Node Syndrome

Mucocutaneous lymph node syndrome (MLNS), previously termed Kawasaki's disease, occurs mostly in children and is characterized by erythematous changes involving the skin and mucous membranes. Diagnostic criteria have been established (Table 19.5). Additionally, there is a remarkable association, in about a quarter of patients, between MLNS and vasculitis of the coronary vessels.

The skin and mucosal lesions generally resolve without sequelae; however, coronary artery and myocardial involvement may lead to aneurysmal dilatation and eventually to vessel thrombosis. Aspirin and intravenous gamma globulin, administered early in the course, is effective in reducing detectable coronary artery lesions.

Henoch-Schönlein Purpura

Henoch-Schönlein purpura (HSP) often presents acutely with:
- A skin rash
- Joint complaints
- Abdominal pain
- Sometimes, renal dysfunction.

19

TABLE 19.5 — DIAGNOSTIC GUIDELINES OF MUCOCUTANEOUS LYMPH NODE SYNDROME

Principal Symptoms
- Fever lasting from 1 to 2 weeks and not responding to antibiotics
- Bilateral congestion of ocular conjunctivae
- Changes of lips and oral cavity:
  - Dryness, redness and fissuring of lips
  - Protuberance of tongue papillae (strawberry-tongue)
  - Diffuse reddening of oral and pharyngeal mucosa
- Changes of peripheral extremities:
  - Reddening of palms and soles (initial stage)
  - Indurative edema (initial stage)
  - Membranous desquamation from fingertips (convalescent stage)
- Polymorphous exanthema of body trunk without vesicles or crusts
- Acute nonpurulent swelling of cervical lymph nodes of 1.5 cm or more in diameter

Other Significant Symptoms or Findings
- Carditis, especially myocarditis and pericarditis
- Diarrhea
- Arthralgia or arthritis
- Proteinuria and increase of leukocytes in urine sediment
- Changes in blood tests:
  - Leukocytes with shift to the left
  - Slight decrease in erythrocyte and hemoglobin levels
  - Increased ESR
  - Positive CRP
  - Increased α_2-globulin
  - Negative ASLO
- Changes occasionally observed:
  - Aseptic meningitis
  - Mild jaundice or slight increase of serum transaminase

Abbreviations: ESR, erythrocyte sedimentation rate; CRP, C-reactive protein; ASLO, anti-streptolysin–O.

The skin rash, often palpable purpura at the waist or below, is one of the most common features of HSP. Other common rashes seen with HSP are urticaria, petechiae and erythema multiforme. The ankles and knees are the most commonly involved, and periarticular swelling accounts for the physical findings. Abdominal pain, thought to be due to mesenteric vasculitis, is generally cramping in quality; hemoccult testing is often positive. Gross bleeding from the gastrointestinal tract does occur, but is unusual. The abdominal pain may be of sufficient severity to suggest a need for surgical intervention; however, in most cases, this is not necessary. The presence of the skin rash and joint pain are helpful in guiding the evaluation.

In most, this syndrome is transient and resolves over several weeks. Prognosis often is directly related to the presence and extent of renal disease. Detected clinically as hematuria (which may be gross), renal involvement can include a rapidly progressive glomerulonephritis, leading to renal failure.

Other organ involvement is more unusual, but central nervous system and pulmonary vasculitis may at times dominate the clinical picture.

In many, supportive care is all that is necessary. Those with renal disease, altered sensorium, or other organ-threatening complications are often treated more vigorously with corticosteroids and other agents, but this is empiric.

Cryoglobulinemia

Cryoglobulins are immunoglobulin (Ig) molecules that become insoluble when they are cooled below body temperature. They are divided into three classes:
- Type 1, which are monoclonal antibodies, usually IgM, that are found in hematological ma-

lignancies such as Waldenström's macroglobulinemia

- Type II, which are monoclonal rheumatoid factors that interact with IgG
- Type III, which are polyclonal rheumatoid factors that bind to IgG.

Type II cryoglobulins are seen in patients with lymphoproliferative disorders and certain rheumatic disorders such as rheumatoid arthritis. The development of serology to hepatitis C has led researchers to recognize that many cases of type II and type III cryoglobulins, previously thought to be "idiopathic," are associated with this virus.

Apart from signs or symptoms due to the underlying disorder associated with the cryoglobulin, the cryoglobulins themselves may not cause symptoms. A sign attributable to cryoglobulins is palpable purpura, which histologically is a leukocytoclastic vasculitis. Peripheral neuropathies and membranoproliferative glomerulonephritis due to vasculitis are also seen in some symptomatic patients.

Treatment is generally focused on the underlying disorder. Many patients with asymptomatic cryoglobulinemia may need no treatment. Alternatively, those with renal or neurological disease are often treated empirically with corticosteroids, alkylating agents, or plasmapheresis.

Thromboangiitis Obliterans

Commonly known as Buerger's disease, it is a vascular disorder seen in tobacco users, particularly with cigarette use. Symptoms are generally those of extremity ischemia, but frequently occur in younger males, particularly those under 50 or 60 years of age. Claudication, Raynaud's disease, and ischemic ulcers are among the more common signs and symptoms.

Histological evaluations have demonstrated an inflammatory infiltrate in the biopsied vessels. Measures designed to limit inflammation have not been successful. Complete abstinence from tobacco is successful in most.

SUGGESTED READING

Arend WP, Michel BA, Bloch DA, et al. The American College of Rheumatology 1990 criteria for the classification of Takayasu arteritis. *Arthritis Rheum.* 1990;33:1129-1134.

Calabrese LH, Michel BA, Bloch DA, et al. The American College of Rheumatology 1990 criteria for the classification of hypersensitivity vasculitis. *Arthritis Rheum.* 1990;33:1108-1113.

International Study Group for Behçets Disease. Criteria for diagnosis of Behçet's Disease. *Lancet.* 1990;335:1078-1080.

Kawasaki T, Kosaki F, Okawa S, Shigematsu I, Yanagawa H. A new infanile acute febrile mucocutaneous lymph node syndrome (MLNS) prevailing in Japan. *Pediatrics.* 1974;54:271-276.

Leavitt RY, Fauci AS, Bloch DA, et al. The American College of Rheumatology 1990 criteria for the classification of Wegener's granulomatosis. *Arthritis Rheum.* 1990;33:1101-1107.

Lightfoot RW Jr, Michel BA, Bloch DA, et al. The American of Rheumatology 1990 criteria for the classification of polyarteritis nodosa. *Arthritis Rheum.* 1990;33:1088-1093.

Masi AT, Hunder GG, Lie JT, et al. The American College of Rheumatology 1990 criteria for the classification of Churg-Strauss syndrome (allergic granulomatosis and angiitis). *Arthritis Rheum.* 1990;33:1094-1100.

Mill JA, Michel BA, Bloch DA, et al. The American College of Rheumatology 1990 criteria for the classification of Henoch-Schönlein purpura. *Arthritis Rheum.* 1990;33:1114-1121.

19

20   Resources

American Academy of Orthopaedic Surgeons (AAOS)
6300 N. River Road
Rosemont, IL 60018-4262
Phone: 847/823-7186 or 800/346-AAOS
Fax: 847/823-8125
Website: www.aaos.org

The AAOS provides education and practice management services for orthopaedic surgeons and allied health professionals. Founded as a nonprofit organization in 1933, the Academy has grown to service about 20,000 members internationally; it is the world's largest medical association of musculoskeletal specialists.

American Academy of Physical Medicine and Rehabilitation (AAPM&R)
Suite 2500
One IBM Plaza
Chicago, IL 60611-3604
Phone: 312/464-9700
Fax: 312/464-0227
Website: www.aapmr.org

The AAPM&R is the national medical society representing 5600 physicians who are specialists in the field of physical medicine and rehabilitation. They care for patients with acute and chronic pain, including musculoskeletal problems like back pain and fibromyalgia.

20

**American Autoimmune Related Diseases
Association, Inc. (AARDA)**
15475 Gratiot Avenue
Detroit, MI 48205
Phone: 313/371-8600
Literature requests: 800/598-4668
Website: www.aarda.org

AARDA is dedicated to the eradication of autoimmune diseases, the alleviation of suffering, and the socioeconomic impact of autoimmunity through fostering and facilitating collaboration in the areas of education, research and patient services in an effective, ethical and efficient manner.

**American Association for
Chronic Fatigue Syndrome (AACFS)**
c/o Harborview Medical Center
325 Ninth Avenue
Box 359780
Seattle, WA 98104
Phone: 206/521-1932
Fax: 206/521-1930
Website: weber.u.washington.edu/~dedra/aacfs1.html

AACFS is a nonprofit organization of research scientists, physicians, licensed medical health-care professionals, and other individuals and institutions interested in promoting the stimulation, coordination, and exchange of ideas for CFS research and patient care, as well as providing periodic reviews of current clinical, research and treatment ideas on CFS for the benefit of CFS patients and others. Topics include CFS and fibromyalgia, among others.

American College of Rheumatology (ACR)
Suite 250
1800 Century Place
Atlanta, GA 30345
www.rheumatology.org

The ACR is an organization of physicians, health professionals, and scientists that serves its members through programs of education, research and advocacy which foster excellence in the care of people with arthritis and rheumatic and musculoskeletal diseases. The web site includes a list of publications and rheumatology links.

American Juvenile Arthritis Organization (AJAO)
1330 West Peachtree Street
Atlanta, GA 30309
Phone: 404/872-7100
Website: www.arthritis.org/ajao

The AJAO serves as an advocate and works to improve the quality of life for children with rheumatic diseases and their families, specifically by working toward improved medical care, providing collective and individual advocacy, stimulating research, and providing education and support.

American Lyme Disease Foundation, Inc. (ALDF)
293 Route 100
Somers, NY 10589
Phone: 914/277-6970
Fax: 941/277-6974
Website: www.aldf.com

ALDF supports research and plays a key role in providing reliable and scientifically accurate information to the public and health-care providers. The information on Lyme disease presented in this website has been reviewed, approved and partially funded by the Centers for Disease Control and Prevention.

American Occupational Therapy Association, Inc.
(AOTA)
4720 Montgomery Lane
Bethesda, MD 20814-3425
Phone: 301/652-2682
Fax: 301/652-7711
Website: www.aota.org

AOTA advances occupational therapy as the pre-eminent profession in promoting the health, productivity and quality of life of individuals and society through the therapeutic application of occupational tasks.

Arthritis and Rheumatism International (ARI)
1330 West Peachtree Street
Atlanta, GA 30309
Website: www.arthritis.org/connections/international/

ARI is an association of national lay organizations whose members are principally people whose lives are affected by arthritis and whose activities are volunteer based. ARI's aim is to provide a forum for the worldwide exchange of knowledge and experiences among organizations of people affected by arthritis and to strengthen their voices through worldwide co-operation.

Arthritis Canada
Website: www.arthritis.ca

Arthritis Canada is the effort of a dedicated team of arthritis health-care providers and volunteers. It was developed so that people with arthritis, their fami-

276

lies and caregivers could find a reliable and comprehensive source of information. Website encompasses several organizations.

Arthritis Foundation
1330 West Peachtree Street
Atlanta, GA 30309
404/872-7100
Website: www.arthritis.org
Arthritis Answers Line: 800/283-7800

The mission of the Arthritis Foundation is to support research to find the cure for and prevention of arthritis and to improve the quality of life for those affected by arthritis. Website includes information about the *Arthritis Today* publication, news and facts, research resources, resource room, along with links to related websites.

Arthritis Today
Website: www.arthritis.org/at

Arthritis Today is the No. 1 magazine for people who have arthritis and for those who care about someone who does. It is published 6 times a year by the Arthritis Foundation.

Fibromyalgia Wellness Letter
Website: www.arthritis.org/resource/newsletters/
fibro_wellness.shtml

From the publishers of *Arthritis Today* comes a new publication, *Fibromyalgia Wellness Letter*. This essential newsletter is packed with all the latest information, reliable advice and up-to-date research news about fibromyalgia, the second–most-commonly diagnosed musculoskeletal disorder.

20

Arthritis National Research Foundation
Suite 440
200 Oceangate
Long Beach, CA 90802
Phone: 800/588-CURE (2873)
Website: www.curearthritis.org

Arthritis National Research Foundation's primary purpose is to provide financial support to research studies aimed at discovering new knowledge for the prevention, treatment and cure of arthritis and other rheumatic diseases.

CliniWeb
Website: www.ohsu.edu/cliniweb

CliniWeb is an index and table of contents to clinical information on the World Wide Web. It now has direct links to MedLine searches via the PubMed system at the National Library of Medicine.

HealthWorld Online
Website: www.healthy.net

This website provides information on many diseases, including musculoskeletal disorders.

Kids on the Block, Inc.
9385-C Gerwig Lane
Columbia, MD 21046-1583
Phone: 800/368-KIDS (5437) or 410/290-9095
Fax: 410/290-9358
Website: www.kotb.com

The purpose of the Kids on the Block is to provide educational puppet programs which enlighten all children on the issues of disability awareness, medical education differences, and social concerns. Program topics include children with arthritis among other health-related issues.

Lupus Canada
Website: www.lupuscanada.org

This site is provided as a source of information about Lupus Canada, its member organizations, lupus the disease, as well as activities of interest to people with lupus, their families and friends.

Lupus Foundation of America, Inc.
Website: internet-plaza.net/lupus; also
                www.hamline.edu/lupus

Website lists information on government advocacy, commonly asked questions about lupus, current information on lupus, and a research and resource library.

The Lyme Disease Network
43 Winton Road
East Brunswick, NJ 08816
Website: www.lymenet.org

Publishers of the *LymeNet Newsletter* designed to present readers with up-to-date developments, including new treatment protocols, research news, and political events. The newsletter is free to anyone with an internet e-mail address.

Mayo Health Oasis
Website: www.mayohealth.org

This website, sponsored by the Mayo Foundation for Medical Education and Research, has a wealth of information on many of the musculoskeletal disorders.

MedWeb
Website: www.gen.emory.edu/medweb/
  medweb.rheumatology.html

This website has information on many rheumatology topics such as ankylosing spondylitis, arthritis, fibromyalgia, Lyme disease, polymyalgia rheumatica, scleroderma, and more. It also provides links to other rheumatology websites.

The Merck Manual
Website: www.merck.com

Chapters from *The Merck Manual* can be viewed at this website.

Multipurpose Arthritis and Musculoskeletal Diseases Centers
Website: www.arthritis.org/connections/maamdc.shtml

This website has a state-by-state listing of multipurpose arthritis and musculoskeletal diseases centers, including addresses and phone/fax numbers.

Myositis Association of America (MAA)
1420 Huron Court
Harrisonburg, VA 22801
Phone: 540/433-7686
Fax: 540/432-0206
Website: www.myositis.org

The MAA is a nonprofit organization committed to helping people with inflammatory myopathies through a variety of information and support services. Information is available on polymyositis, dermatomyositis, inclusion body myositis, and juvenile myositis.

**National Fibromyalgia Research
Association (NFRA)**
PO Box 500
Salem, OR 97302
Website: www.teleport.com/~nfra/Nfraintr.htm

This organization is dedicated to education, treatment and finding a cure for fibromyalgia. Since its inception in 1992, its members have built on this premise politically, financially and educationally in an effort to raise public, medical and government awareness of this debilitating disease.

**National Institute of Arthritis and
Musculoskeletal and Skin Diseases (NIAMS)**
National Institutes of Health
Bethesda, MD 20892-2350
Website: www.nih.gov/niams

NIAMS is one component of the National Institutes of Health. NIAMS conducts and supports basic, clinical and epidemiologic research and training, and disseminates information on many diseases, including many forms of arthritis and diseases of the musculoskeletal system and the skin.

National Psoriasis Foundation (NPF)
Website: www.psoriasis.org

The NPF is a membership organization composed of people who have psoriasis and psoriatic arthritis, their family members, friends, physicians, nurses, researchers and corporations who have united in order to improve the quality of life for people who have psoriasis and psoriatic arthritis, to educate the public about psoriasis, and to support psoriasis research.

20

Scleroderma Foundation
Suite 201
89 Newbury Street
Danvers, MA 01923
Phone: 978/750-4499
Fax: 978/750-9902
Help Line: 800/722-HOPE (4673)
Website: www.scleroderma.org

Website includes information regarding scleroderma research, education and support.

Spondylitis Association of America (SAA)
Website: www.spondylitis.org

The SAA is a national nonprofit organization established in 1983. SAA is dedicated to improving the quality of life of those living with ankylosing spondylitis (AS) and diseases related to AS, such as Reiter's syndrome/reactive arthritis, psoriatic arthritis, spondylitis of inflammatory bowel disease, and undifferentiated spondyloarthropathy.

Systemic Lupus Erythematosus (SLE)
Foundation, Inc.
149 Madison Avenue
New York, NY 10016
Phone: 800/558-0121
Fax: 212/545-1843
Website: www.kumc.edu/gec/support/systemic.html

This site provides links to support groups, national organizations, and information regarding lupus, as well as locations of genetic counselors and clinical geneticists by geographical location.

USA Fibromyalgia Association
Box 1483
Dublin, OH 43017
Phone: 614/675-1152 or 614/851-9177

Fibrositis and fibromyalgia sufferers can find information about the disease and how to live with it.

20

Note: Page numbers in *italics* indicate figures;
page numbers followed by t indicate tables.

285

297